Your Baby's Beginning

A PARENTING GUIDE FOR YOUR BABY'S FIRST WEEK

BY FRANK W. BOWEN, MD

ISBN: 978-1-7336158-7-7

Edited by: Elizabeth Russell and Amy Ashby

PipeVine
P R E S S

Published by PipeVine Press
Charlotte, NC
www.warrenpublishing.net
Printed in the United States

This book is dedicated to the amazing journey babies and their parents make in the first week; may it be a helpful companion.

FOREWORD

It has been an honor to have assisted in over 5,000 births during my forty-year obstetric career. It was humbling to know that my primary role, after years of training, was to minimize trauma to mother and baby by providing a safe environment for one of the most profound events in life. It was gratifying to know that colleagues like Dr. Frank Bowen shared the desire to create a safe and atraumatic environment for our fragile patients as they entered a brave new world, drastically in contrast to the dark, warm, watery, and quiet place they had spent the previous nine months.

We are just beginning to learn how our environment affects the way our genes behave. For example, we now know that exposure during pregnancy to elevated levels of hormones such as cortisol, a stress hormone, can lead to low birthweight and increased risk of diabetes, hypertension, and behavior disorders in adults. Surely, the first week of transitioning from fetus to newborn gives parents the opportunity to enhance a child's ability to learn and adapt, hopefully helping mitigate the harmful effects of stress.

Dr. Bowen is uniquely qualified to write about this critical first week of infancy.

After completing his neonatology fellowship at Children's National Medical Center in Washington, DC, Dr. Bowen became director of neonatology at William Beaumont Hospital in El Paso, Texas.

In 1981, he became director of neonatology at Pennsylvania Hospital while also serving on the faculty at the University of Pennsylvania. While there, Dr. Bowen founded the Pennsylvania chapter of the National Perinatal Association. In addition, he served as president of the National Perinatal Association and was elected a member of the American Pediatric Society and is a member of the American Academy of Pediatrics.

It was about this time I became familiar with some of the over sixty articles he had written, as I was a Penn alumnus also working with the National Perinatal Association. Later in his career, Dr. Bowen received a master's in medical management from Tulane University.

After moving to Hilton Head, South Carolina over seventeen years ago, Dr. Bowen became executive medical director of Volunteers in Medicine, a large free clinic for the medically underserved who live or work on Hilton Head Island. The clear, plain-spoken language used in writing *Your Baby's Beginning* is what you would expect if your grandfather were a pediatrician who had written this book especially for you.

The information Dr. Bowen shares with his audience is insightful and will serve as a valuable tool for any parent or grandparent in helping an infant make this important transition to what will hopefully become a productive and happy life.

Raymond L. Cox, MD, MBA
Executive Director, Volunteers in Medicine
Hilton Head Island, South Carolina

ACKNOWLEDGMENTS

First and foremost, I would like to thank the 20,000 or so parents and infants who taught me so very, very much. Next must come my family: my wife Dottie, a neonatal nurse, executive healthcare leader, and sharp observer; our children; and especially our grandchildren who they have brought into the world. Our children and many others used this book and provided many thoughtful comments.

Next are the tremendous contributors to newborn literature who have given us valuable insights into the medical and behavioral abilities of newborn infants. Indeed, both my professional colleagues and the helpful members of Island Writers Network have graciously provided invaluable advice. I also thank Bill Winn, who did the interior illustrations with great patience and good humor. I also thank my VIM college and academic obstetrician, Dr. Ray Cox, for his Forward and insightful comments on the manuscript. And I must mention that the field of newborn medicine has come miles during the course of my own career. The old days of separating parents and infants are thankfully gone. To my colleagues who read this manual and have suggestions—I welcome them!

Finally, and perhaps most importantly, I thank the Lord, who inspired me to write a manual to help parents.

TABLE OF CONTENTS

INTRODUCTION
A Great Beginning

A whole list of "greats" comes with the act of becoming a parent: the great thrill, the great responsibility, the great heir or heiress, the great cry, love, worry ... I could go on and on and so could you.

Having a baby is indeed, great, and very common. It happens over four million times each year in North America alone. Almost all these parents struggle to "do it right." We certainly did with our infants, and my rounds as a doctor specializing in newborn care brought me daily to parents who were trying to understand their new babies.

In the old days, when mothers stayed in the hospital for up to seven days after giving birth, physicians and nurses had time to discuss the gamut of infant physiology and behavior. Today, stays are down to hours to three days, even after Caesarian delivery. Mothers are discharged before health care providers have a chance to share information about the newborn's behavior, feeding, and physical changes she can expect to see and experience at home.

This first few days as parents and infant is an emotional roller coaster of anxiety and joy. Your baby and you are making the biggest transition ever in your lives. How you start will influence how you continue to care for your baby. This beginning time is the time you establish yourself as a parent.

A User's Guide

Your Baby's Beginning is a user's guide rather than just another baby book. It is a detailed look at the baby's change from fetus to newborn to infant. Further, it gives you the information you need to begin communicating with your newborn. You will be learning what a fantastic person your baby is and how both of you can communicate. It serves to introduce your baby's actions in this first critical week. I describe your baby during the time he is changing rapidly, going from a fetal life in his mother's womb to life as a separate person. At the same time, you and your infant are getting acquainted with each other. As you do, you will establish your own style of parenting and set the tone for a lifetime of interactions between you and your child.

Your Baby's Beginning is interactional, designed to allow both parents to record their observations in detail as their infant changes over the first week. This interactional design is specific because we know that you and your baby are individuals. By recording your interactions, feelings, and questions, you will establish your parenting pattern.

Also, *Your Baby's Beginning* is designed to serve as a bridge to child development that evolves in the months and years to come. I describe the norms to give you a reference point, and more importantly, explain the common variations of normal, the range of differences pediatricians expect to find in healthy babies.

The Arrangement

I will describe variations of normal in three major areas: physical, behavioral, and feeding. I will try to cover the full range of healthy newborns, but there will always be exceptions. A baby who does not match our description may be perfectly fine; however, if you observe something outside of the range we have described, ask your baby's doctor to check it out. I will alert you to situations that signal a need for professional attention, and I will help you get acquainted with your baby and learn what is normal for him.

Also, if you read of differences in other baby and child care books, bring this to your physician's attention. The majority of these differences are what are called "variations of normal," or the use of different terms to describe the same thing, such as "vigorous" and "active."

Your Baby's Beginning is arranged chronologically, showing how your baby, you, and the interaction between the two of you evolves, and how these first interactions are a basis for later parenting. Each chapter begins with an overview and then details three intertwining themes: physical development, behavioral development, and feeding.

In physical development, I trace the changes in your baby's structure and function from the first examination in the delivery room through his full adaptation to life outside your womb. Understanding these changes enables you to recognize his needs and bring your own touch to meeting those needs.

If babies were all physics and chemistry, they would be simple to care for—and no fun at all. But they are fun; from the start, they are vibrant, emotional, responsive people. As we follow their development, we will explore the fascinating world of infant behavior. You shall, I promise, delight in the repertoire of behaviors and responses your infant possesses. You and your baby stimulate and respond to each other. Parenting is your side of the interaction, and I will discuss it as part of behavioral development.

At birth, most babies do not do very much in the eating department. However, within a few days they learn how to eat, and turn into veritable eating machines. How your baby responds to feeding is part physical need, part baby's behavior, and part parent's behavior. I give it a section of its own because of its importance to all of you in the first week.

Of course, no book can answer all your specific questions about your baby. Your pediatrician can, and I urge you to ask about any of your concerns. Parents sometimes hesitate, thinking, perhaps, their questions are silly or that they are taking too much of the doctor's time. But any question lacking an answer is legitimate; you need to understand everything about your baby. In *Your Baby's Beginning*, I give you an introduction to new babies in general. Make sure to ask your doctor about your baby as a unique and special individual.

Most pediatricians today have e-mail or voicemail systems that allow them to easily respond to questions without the need for an office visit.

I will also address some problems infants sometimes have at birth or before. Sadly, not all pregnancies end in joy. Some end in the distress and grief surrounding serious medical issues or even death of the infant. I cover some of these issues in the appropriate sections and the more serious ones in the final chapter of the book, "The Hard Chapter." I urge you to read this chapter even if all has gone well for you, because I can practically guarantee that you will have a friend or relative who is dealing with this tragedy. Your knowledge will help you to be a support to them in their deep distress.

Terminology

At this point, let me clarify terminology concerning medical personnel. You may choose a pediatrician, family practitioner, nurse practitioner, or midwife to supervise your infant's initial health care. Any of these professionals is well qualified to take care of a healthy newborn, but listing them all is cumbersome. We will use primary care provider (PCP) as a general term for the person who provides primary medical care for your baby. In addition, there are people who provide specific types of care, such as lactation consultants, nutritionists, laboratory technicians, and the like. I will refer to them specifically.

You may also encounter many technical medical terms. Generally, I have included a technical term (such as "resuscitated") in parentheses and used the more easily understood term, such as "helped" or "assisted." Your PCP or nurse should be able to clear up any confusion you have.

Also, please bear with me as I delve (hopefully, not too deeply) into the science behind certain events such as temperature regulation, the production of breast milk, and others. I believe that understanding how our bodies work and adapt in this world is important in making logical decisions. Since neither our bodies nor our babies are able to speak, we must have other ways of understanding why things occur the way they do.

A few words, too, about gender: I have chosen to alternate "hes" and "shes" in this book by chapter, because it does not seem right to call babies "its," and the he/she convention is stilted and bothersome.

We should also be clear that although this book may sometimes seem addressed to mothers, it is meant for fathers as well (I am one myself). Parenting, whether you are Mother or Father, begins with sensitivity to your infant's needs. Sensitivity to needs begins with observing and understanding what you observe. Fathers do this as well as mothers. In fact, with the obvious exception of breastfeeding, anything Mom does with the new baby, Dad can do also.

Finally, not all babies are born at exactly one minute after midnight. So, using the terms Day One, Day Two, etc. is meant to give you a perspective. Think of the days as twenty-four hours since birth. Remember, babies do not know about day and night—that is a concept new to them.

Congratulations

New parenthood is exciting, whether it is your first time or your seventh. Each event is so important, you cannot imagine ever forgetting it. Experience, however, tells us that even these memories fade, which is another reason this book has space to record your impressions and observations. We invite and encourage both Mother and Father to make notes about your thoughts so you will have a permanent record of your baby's beginning. I recommend that you fill in some of the questions you may have as you read before delivery. They may be relevant later and you may forget in the business of parenting.

Finally, my best wishes to you and your new baby.

Have a great time getting to know each other.

DAY ZERO
In the Delivery Room

The First Minutes: In the Delivery Room

*T*he moment of birth marks the most dramatic change a person ever makes. As he leaves the safe haven of his mother's body, he must breathe air for the first time. His lungs begin to function, and his blood circulation shifts to rely on lungs rather than the placenta to gain oxygen and remove carbon dioxide. After nine months of relying on his mother for life, he must suddenly adjust to life as a separate person.

The moment a baby is born, his universe changes. He goes from a world that is dark, warm, wet, and quiet to one that is bright, cold, dry, and noisy; from an environment with little sensory stimulation to one with a great array of stimuli to see, hear, touch, taste, and smell.

The past nine months have prepared him for his birth. As a fetus, he is designed to withstand the hard work of labor and delivery. The labor and birth process serve as a signal that triggers a unique physiologic (functional) change that allows his body to operate in a very different way.

While he was a fetus, the baby was getting oxygen from his mother. Mom was literally breathing for two, supplying oxygen to and removing carbon dioxide from her baby's bloodstream and getting him accustomed to having the right amounts of both. That was a big part of the placenta's function.

Then, during labor, he was slightly deprived of oxygen and built up higher levels of carbon dioxide. This may sound like a problem, but this oxygen deprivation is in fact a nicely tuned mechanism that prompts the infant to breathe at the moment of his birth. This shift in the levels of oxygen and carbon dioxide creates his urge to breathe. He has the same feeling you have when you hold your breath for even a minute—try it. Did you feel the building urge to breathe?

The first breaths trigger a shift in circulation known as the change from fetal to adult circulation. The fetus's heart pumps blood to the placenta through the umbilical cord and away from the lungs. Now, that route must be reversed. Delivering the baby and clamping the umbilical cord stops blood flow to and from the placenta; taking air into the lungs, usually through crying, causes the blood vessels in the lungs to open, which allows blood to flow to the lungs. When babies have fetal circulation, they appear blue (cyanotic). As soon as they shift to adult circulation, they suddenly become pink. You may be lucky enough to see this happen in the delivery room—however, it happens quickly, usually in the first minute or two after delivery.

After delivery, your newborn is at the center of a swirl of activity, all designed to watch and help him if he needs it. He is taking responsibility for breathing, pumping blood around his tiny body, regulating his body temperature, and maintaining other vital functions. WOW—such a bunch to do in just a few minutes!

Most babies accomplish this task by themselves. Occasionally, a baby needs assistance to start breathing. In this case, the PCP caring for your baby will explain what has been done and if any further treatment is needed.

If your baby needs assistance with breathing, you may feel quite anxious during the time that he is being helped (resuscitated). This feeling is natural and normal and part of the beginning of parenthood. The sound of your infant's cry after successful assistance will immediately replace anxiety with joy. Parenthood can be a roller coaster experience.

APGAR Scores

Within seconds of your baby's birth, your baby will be examined and rated on a scale of zero to ten. The rating is called the *APGAR score* after Dr. Virginia Apgar, the doctor who devised the test. The first APGAR score, at one minute, measures how well the infant has handled labor and delivery. The second score, done at five minutes, tells how well he is breathing and doing on his own.

The APGAR score is the sum of scores for five different factors: color, breathing, muscle tone, reaction to a stimulus (reflex irritability), and heartbeat. Each factor receives a score of zero, one, or two. Color, for example, is scored as zero if the baby is pale, one if he is blue, and two if he is pink.

For breathing, a baby who is not breathing gets a zero, irregular breathing gets a one, and active crying a two.

In scoring muscle tone, a baby who is limp gets zero. Flexing of arms and legs gets a one, and active movement a two.

We measure reflex irritability by pacing a catheter (a very fine tube) in the baby's nose. If the baby does not react, the score is zero. A grimace gets a one, and a vigorous protest results in a score of two. I would get a two on this one—would you?

The heartbeat is counted and scored as zero if there is no heartbeat, one if the rate is less than one hundred per minute, and two if it is greater than one hundred per minute.

A one-minute APGAR score of seven to ten indicates the baby is doing very well. A score of four to six means that the baby is having slight difficulty and needs some assistance. Three or less indicates a significant problem. A low APGAR score is a matter of concern. However, there is not a solid correlation between the APGAR score and subsequent development. Your baby's PCP will discuss any issues related to a need for resuscitation. Here is a table to write your baby's APGAR scores.

	One Minute	Five Minute	Comments
Color			
Breathing			
Muscle Tone			
Reflex Irritability			
Heart Beat			
Total			

Other Delivery Room Activities

In addition to examining and scoring your baby, a PCP or nurse may administer eye drops and a vitamin K injection, and will place bands that identify the baby as yours.

The eye drops are used because bacteria present in the birth canal can cause eye infections in newborns. Vitamin K is needed for normal blood clotting. It is one of the family of vitamins (A, D, E, and K) that do not dissolve in water. These vitamins do not cross the placenta well, so newborns may be low in these vitamins. Early breastfeeding provides ample amounts of A, D and E, but not so much K. Children and adults use bacteria in their intestines to make vitamin K. It takes a few days for bacteria to establish residence in the baby's intestine (see—not all bacteria are bad), so the dose given in the delivery room is designed to tide him over until he has a supply of his own. Without the vitamin K, the baby might develop a serious disease called *hemorrhagic disease of the newborn.* Thanks to the injection, we rarely see this disease today.

Identifying the baby includes putting his footprints and the mother's thumbprint on the same form. You and your baby will also have identically numbered bracelets. Nurses will check these bracelets if there is any time you and your baby are separated during your hospital or birthing center stay.

In many birthing situations today, you have already been holding, cuddling, and feeding your baby during all this identification activity. Whatever the setting, this is the time to hold each other: Mother, Father, and baby. Do not worry about exams or feeding—just enjoy being a family.

Your Impressions:

APGAR scores are important in evaluating your baby's health and his ability to function in our world, but they are not the stuff of parents' fond memories. Having recorded the score, here is a chance to write down your own first impressions … what was important to you when you first saw your new little son or daughter?

1. What was your very first impression?

2. What are your questions?

3. What was reassuring to you?

4. What caused you to worry or be anxious?

5. What raised questions or caused you to wonder?

6. Is your baby different from what you expected? How?

7. Describe your baby.

Here is a spot for a photo of your new family.

DAY ONE
A Day of Recovery

Overview

The intensity and excitement of labor and delivery are over. You and your baby are recovering from the experience of birth and adapting to the immense changes.

Both parents are beginning their new roles, but it is the smallest member of the family who is making the biggest adjustment. Her most abrupt change came in the delivery room, where she had to quickly adjust from being a fetus to a newborn. Now she must experience and respond to the world around her.

The physical evaluation of your newborn is one of the most important events in the first day. This first examination addresses the questions and concerns about whether the new baby is normal. As I describe healthy newborns in the section on Physical Changes, I will introduce you to many of the differences (individual variations) that make each baby unique—indeed, the same as those that make each of us different.

Behavioral changes are less obvious during the first day. In the past, babies were thought of as creatures who sleep, eat, and do little else. Now we understand that infants arrive with a full repertoire of behaviors, and the first day is not too early to observe and begin to understand them.

Feeding barely begins on day one. As I shall explain, babies are born "pre-fed" and don't need to eat much for the first few days.

Nursing at this stage, whether from breast or bottle, is a time for learning how to feed, a time to enjoy your baby and not worry about how much she is taking.

Physical Changes

Sometime during the first day, your baby's PCP will perform a thorough physical examination. If your PCP attended the delivery, he performed the exam in the delivery room along with the APGAR scoring. Often, a nurse does the preliminary exam, leaving the PCP to do the complete physical in your room. Either way, the complete examination should be done within the first twenty-four hours following birth.

Preliminary Examination

The PCP or nurse who does the preliminary exam will take your baby's temperature, pulse, and breathing rate and look her over to evaluate her general state of health. He will also perform an assessment of gestational age (the length of time that the baby has been growing since conception).

While you were pregnant, your PCP estimated the duration of your pregnancy. He used criteria such as the date of your last menstrual period, the date when you first felt the baby moving, the size of your uterus and, perhaps, an ultrasound test.

Now that your baby is born, the nurse or PCP has new measures to complete the exam. He can measure the baby's size and evaluate her physical development and nervous system function. Using these measures, he can compute a maturity score that is related to gestational age.

These determinations of size and gestational age are important because they identify babies who have a higher risk of developing problems and require special observation for the first few days. If your baby needs this extra attention, your PCP will take actions that he will explain to you. These actions may require modifying some of the activities described in this book. Such changes should not separate you from your baby. A significant part of this assessment includes the baby's measurements. Here is a chart to record them. The percentile means where on the spectrum of normal your baby's measurements fall compared to the overall population of newborn infants. For instance, a seven-pound girl at forty weeks gestation may be in the fiftieth percentile. Your PCP can explain percentile measures.

Your Baby's Measurements	Measurement	Percentile
Weight		
Length		
Head Circumference		
Gestational Age		

Variations of Normal

Before I describe the features you can observe on your baby, I need to explain the concept of variations of normal. These are the normal differences that are seen from one individual to another. Each of us has certain characteristics that set us apart from other people. Rather than being a sign of any abnormality, these traits are simply variations of normal. They form our individuality. Some of us have blue eyes, some brown, some babies have lots of hair and some are almost bald—all are okay.

As you look at your baby and compare her to other babies, you may note that she, too, is different from the "norm." In practically every case, what you are looking at will be a perfectly healthy variation of normal and no cause for concern. As I go through the physical exam, I will describe and illustrate many of these variations. As you examine your baby, take note of how she differs, of what makes her unique.

If you are concerned or uncertain about any of the variations you observe, ask your PCP. Discussing your observations and thoughts gives you an opportunity to learn and to develop your skills at observing your child. The term "normal" is very broad!

Nursery Routine

If your baby's initial care is in a hospital nursery, the nurses will do an assessment and continue to watch your baby closely during her first hours. Alert to the even most subtle changes, they can spot a potential problem early enough to keep it from developing into a serious difficulty. If you have delivered in an LDRP (Labor-Delivery-Recovery-Postpartum) or a birthing center room, these stabilization procedures will occur in your presence. Regardless of the setting, this observation time is an important time for your baby.

Both hospitals and birthing centers usually have routines for babies during the first few hours after their birth. These provide important precautions for your baby. The observation period usually coincides with the time you need to get cleaned up and settled. Most often, by the time you are ready to have your baby with you, she is ready to be there. In a birthing center, the nurse midwife often does the observation and exam, with PCP backup. Although the setting is different from a hospital nursery, the observation, measurement, and testing should be done in a similar manner.

There is a space below to record the names of the people who helped you at this time.

Pregnancy PCP	
Baby PCP	
Certified Nurse Midwife	
Registered Nurses	
Lactation Consultant	
Other	

The Physical Examination

The complete physical examination of a new baby, or an adult, for that matter, involves observation, palpation, and auscultation. In other words, the PCP looks, feels, and listens.

Observation (looking) is perhaps the most important of the three. PCPs learn to look quickly, to observe many things about a baby in a short time. As I describe each step of the physical exam, I will explain how you can make many of the same observations yourself.

The Baby's Proportions

It seems obvious that babies are not just miniature adults, but nowhere is this more apparent than in the proportions and contours of their bodies. Their heads appear large, about one-fourth of the entire body length, and they look like they have no necks.

The size of the head reflects the fact that it is the most fully developed part of the newborn's body. The brain and cranial nerves are more mature than other organs and systems at the time of birth. I will describe brain function in more detail in the section on neurologic examination.

You don't need a book about newborns to know that the brain is crucial for survival. But did you ever think the face also plays an essential role? It does. An infant does most of her communicating with her face. She signals you with her crying, but she really interacts with you by means of her facial expressions. And interacting with her parents is one of an infant's survival skills.

The head and face are also the most sensitive parts of your baby's body—handling them may make her fussy. Therefore, PCPs usually wait until the end of the physical to examine the baby's face.

Your baby's chest is flat, while her abdomen protrudes. Her legs are small, and usually, quite bowed. (If your baby was born in a breech position, her legs may seem long and extended.)

Whatever her proportions, your new infant is symmetrical, both in structure and in the way she moves. Newborns usually do not move just one arm or one leg at a time. When they go into motion, it is usually with both sides of the body at once, waving both arms or kicking both legs, often in a somewhat random manner.

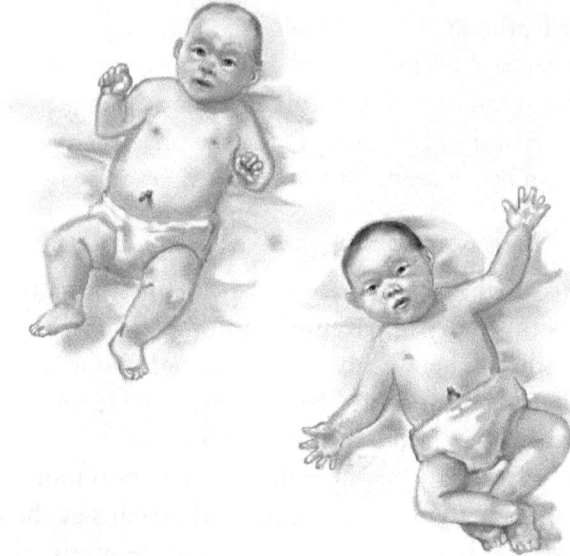

The PCP's first step in examining an infant is undressing the baby and looking at her skin.

At birth, the baby's skin was covered with a white cheesy material called *vernix*. You may have seen it in the delivery room. It is rapidly absorbed or washed off after the baby is born. No one is quite sure exactly what purpose the vernix serves, but its slipperiness suggests that it eases the baby's passage through the birth canal. It also may protect the baby's skin in the liquid environment of the uterus. In either case, after babies are born, they stop making vernix.

By the time she is being examined in the nursery, a newborn's skin is generally pink and smooth. The shade varies in different parts of the body. The face is the palest, the ears and genitals are the darkest. Asian and African American babies have a darker pink undertone to their skin, but their color at birth is lighter than it will be later. All infants' skin takes about six months to develop its permanent color.

Six months is also the length of time it usually takes for what are known as *Mongolian spots* to disappear. These are bluish-black areas on the back and buttocks that many infants have at birth. The spots fade away and are of no significance.

Other spots, birthmarks, are usually variations of normal. Nonetheless, if you have a question about any marks on your baby, call them to your PCP's attention.

Here is a space to describe any birthmarks you find on your baby and to place a picture to aid your memory in years to come. You may really need it if you want to remember, because most birthmarks go away by themselves.

1. Your thoughts.

2. PCP comments?

Here is a spot for a photo of your new baby.

The appearance of a baby's skin changes in response to changes in the temperature of the environment. After nine months in the warmth of the uterus, a newborn needs time to perfect her temperature control. For the first few days, while her temperature regulating system is still learning how to do its job, exposure to a cool temperature will make her skin appear mottled. Her hands and feet may even turn blue. Both are perfectly normal, healthy reactions that will vanish with time.

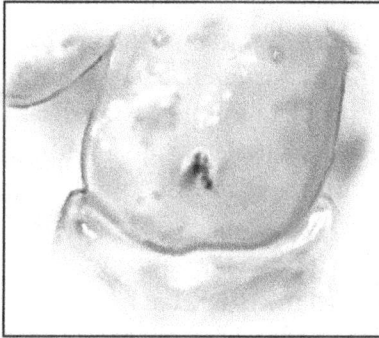

While inspecting your infant's skin, the doctor will also take note of creases on her body. They show up on the arms, backs of the legs, and the feet. As a rule, the creases are symmetrical from side to side. It is especially important to check the leg creases for symmetry; asymmetry here might be a sign of a dislocated hip that would need to be corrected.

The Chest

Having looked at your baby's general contours, her PCP will move on to examine her chest. He will examine the nipple tissue, since its size is related to gestational age. Some babies have supernumerary (extra) nipples on the lower chest or upper abdomen. These tend to fade away and rarely develop into breasts.

Next, your PCP will feel the baby's collar bones. Sometimes one of these bones breaks during delivery. Your delivery PCP or midwife may even have had to break it to deliver your baby if she was very large. Either way, a broken collar bone is rarely a serious matter; it normally heals without any special attention. You need only hold her gently and let nature take its course. Sometimes a figure-eight gauze bandage is used during the healing process. Your nurse will show you how to apply such a dressing.

As he is observing the general contour of your baby's chest, the PCP also watches the rhythmic movement of her ribs as she breathes in and out. Your baby does this at a rate of forty to sixty times per minute. Early on you may notice that the skin between the ribs pulls in a little bit with each breath. This is called *retraction*. It reflects the extra work the baby is doing to rid her lungs of the fluid that filled them in the uterus. Babies take a few hours to clear their lungs. If you notice retractions after that time, tell a PCP or nurse about it. It may be a signal of a lung problem that needs medical attention.

After looking, the PCP will listen to the sound of the baby's breathing. Heard through a stethoscope, breath sounds are clear and equal on both sides of the chest. Sometimes you can hear a vibrating sound in the neck. It is caused by mucus formation and is not a problem.

The PCP will listen to the front, back, and both sides of the chest. If the sounds aren't exactly right, he may continue to observe the baby and listen again within a few hours. Most of the time, what he is hearing is a healthy variation of normal, due to something as insignificant as mucus or the position of the baby's head. If the sounds are still not right when he rechecks the baby's lungs, he may request a chest x-ray and other tests to determine if a problem is developing.

While listening to the chest, the PCP pauses a bit over the left side to listen to the heartbeat. Now you may see a demonstration of soothing techniques as the PCP politely asks your baby to stop crying for a minute so he can hear her heart sounds.

The sounds come from blood flowing through the valves that separate the chambers of the heart as it pumps blood to the lungs and the body. As you recall, your baby's circulation changed dramatically at birth.

While the baby was in the uterus, a special fetal blood vessel called the *ductus arteriosus* moved blood away from the lungs as the placenta was providing oxygen. The lungs were full of amniotic fluid while she was a fetus. Now this vessel must close; a normal process that takes a few days. During this time, your baby's PCP may hear a murmur, an extra sound created by blood flowing through the ductus as it closes. Other conditions, some significant, some not, can also cause murmurs. If the PCP hears a murmur when he listens to your baby's heart, he will do a more thorough evaluation, including checking pulses and blood pressure in different parts of the body. This is another example of the importance of repeated observation in evaluating a changing infant. If there is any question, he may do additional tests such as an electrocardiogram (EKG), ultrasound, or chest X-ray.

It's only natural for you to be concerned if your baby has a murmur. I can tell you, in general, that the majority of murmurs are not significant. They either go away as the baby develops or are considered "functional" or "innocent," a kind of variation of normal.

A small minority of murmurs are caused by structural abnormalities that require medical attention but, in most cases, will not prevent you from taking your baby home and enjoying her normal development. Your PCP will arrange for any special follow-up that may be needed. He will also explain any precautions that you need to take.

The Abdomen

The PCP now moves down the baby's body to examine her belly. It looks like a soft round hill, crowned by the umbilical cord. At birth, the cord was clear. Within an hour or so the cord turned white and firm. You can see the line between the cord and the skin at the spot where the cord is attached to the abdomen.

The cord attachment site is actually a hole in the abdominal wall. During the seven to ten days it takes for the skin to grow completely over this hole, the cord remains attached as a kind of plug. When it is no longer needed, the cord falls away.

Sometimes the diameter of the cord and the hole it covers are so large that the umbilicus protrudes, looking like a hernia pouch. It may stay that way for six months or a year, until the strengthening abdominal muscles close the hole. This is another normal variation that does not require any treatment unless it starts to grow larger or persists past a year. Bellybands, by the way, will not prevent these umbilical hernias.

After looking, the PCP feels the baby's abdomen to check the size of the liver, spleen, and kidneys. This part of the exam, too, may start your baby fussing and give you another chance to observe soothing techniques in action.

The Back

Your PCP has probably looked at the baby's back while listening to your baby's lungs. In addition to checking for Mongolian spots, he looks closely at the area just above the buttocks crack. Some babies have a depression there, which may or may not be hairy, called a *pilonidal dimple*. Usually the only significance of a pilonidal dimple is that it requires extra attention when you bathe your baby. Most of them flatten out as the baby grows. Occasionally, though, a pilonidal dimple is a sign of spina bifida, an abnormality of the spine. Should this be the case, you will need to discuss the situation with your baby's PCP to find out just how serious the situation is and what needs to be done.

The Genitals

The PCP will begin this part of the exam, for both boy and girl babies, by palpating the groin area to check for signs of a hernia. This is one time when it is helpful for the baby to cry. Crying increases the pressure within her abdomen and makes a hernia more visible as a bulge in the groin area. Hernias are more common in pre-term than in full-term infants. This type of hernia, unlike the umbilical type, does require surgical correction. If you notice a bulge in your baby's groin, show it to a nurse or PCP.

The groin is a convenient place to feel a baby's pulse. PCPs often check it while examining this portion of the anatomy. You might want to try it, too, not to look for any problem but simply because it's interesting. To feel the pulse, put your finger halfway between the genitals and the hip in the fold where the leg attaches to the body.

Male Genitals

An infant boy's genitals should appear well-developed, looking like a miniature of an adult's. His penis is about one inch long, although chubbiness or a large scrotum may make it appear shorter. More often, the scrotum will look small. This is especially true if your son has been undressed and cool for a while, as this part of his body, too, is sensitive to the surrounding temperature. (By the way, babies do get erections, which are usually a sign they are about to urinate.)

Regardless of the size of the scrotum, it should be possible to feel two testicles within it, each about the size of a large peanut. There are two conditions of which you should be aware. Both require watching and both usually correct themselves with time. The first, a hydrocele, is an accumulation of fluid around the testicle, making it feel larger than normal. It does no harm to the testicle but will need to be watched to be sure that it clears up properly.

The second condition is an undescended testicle (or testicles). These glands start out in the abdomen and gradually move down to the scrotum late in gestation. Sometimes one or both have not yet reached the scrotum at birth. You may be able to feel it or see it as a little bump resembling a hernia. In most cases, the testicle will move into its normal position and observation is all that is required.

The baby's penis seems to come to a point of foreskin. At this stage, there are bits of tissue connecting the foreskin to the penis and making it difficult to retract the foreskin. If the baby is not circumcised, these "bridges" will go away over the next few months and you will be able to retract the foreskin. Until then, there is no need to force it back. The tip of the foreskin may have small glandular accumulations that look like pimples. They will go away quickly.

If your son is circumcised, this skin will be removed. I will discuss circumcision and the decision about it in some detail in the chapter on day two.

Female Genitals

Newborn girls' genitalia look different from adult women's. The outer skin folds, called *labia majora,* are separated and the inner folds, the *labia minora,* are prominent and red in color. This difference is even more conspicuous in premature infants. The clitoris, the bit of tissue at the top of the labia minora, is usually large in comparison to adult proportions.

Some baby girls have a small protrusion in the vagina. This is a hymeneal skin tag that will regress with time. You may also notice, by the end of the first day, a white vaginal discharge. This, too, is normal and no cause for concern.

Stools and Hygiene

I digress for a moment from the physical examination. Since the baby's diaper is removed for this part of the exam, it may be an opportune moment to observe her stool. Sometime during the first day, the baby will have her first bowel movement. For a day or two, with almost every feeding, she will be passing a dark greenish-black, sticky substance called *meconium.* This material accumulated in her intestine during pregnancy.

When she passes the meconium and, later, stools, the genital area will need to be cleaned. This is a sensitive part of the body, so you will want to be gentle and thorough in cleansing it. The best procedure to use is described in the section on bathing.

The Legs and Feet

A newborn's legs are much shorter, compared to the size of her body, than those of an adult. They bend inward because of the way they were folded in your uterus. In time, as she begins to stand and support her own weight, her legs will straighten out.

As part of the physical exam, the PCP will check your infant's muscle tone by pulling on her legs and watching her pull them back. He will also check her hips by grasping her knees and rotating them outward.

A newborn's feet look too big for her legs. They are, indeed, almost as long as her lower leg. Her ankles are surrounded by a bunch of normal creases. Her toes are complete, but the nails may be almost invisible. Frequently, one toe overlaps another but will straighten with time. The lower leg is also bent inward. She had to do this to fit inside you. Many of these changes are what we call positional, but will change as she gets used to the world. The lower legs, however, may wait until she begins to stand in about nine months or so.

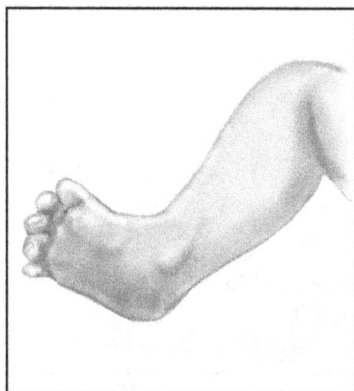

If you compare the form of your baby's foot to your own, you will probably notice that she has no arches. Have no concern about flat feet—she will develop arches later.

If the baby's feet turn in, your PCP will try to straighten them out. Should they not straighten easily, he will recheck them in another day or two and again, if need be, in a couple of weeks. The majority of "bent feet" straighten out on their own. If they don't, there is plenty of time to fix the problem before she needs her feet for balance or movement.

Extreme cases of club foot are exceptions to this rule. These babies must have a cast put on early to correct the problem satisfactorily. In the unlikely event your baby needs a cast, you can discuss the matter with your PCP.

The Arms and Hands

Newborns' arms are well-formed—symmetrical and nicely muscled. If you look closely, you will see symmetrical creases along them. The tiny hands hold a special fascination, perfect miniatures of what they will be.

An infant holds her hand in a fist with the thumb tucked inside the fingers most of the time. If you gently stroke the back of her hand she will open it, revealing all the creases she will ever have.

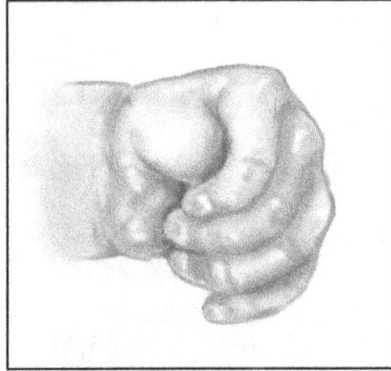

Unlike her almost invisible toenails, a newborn's fingernails are long and sharp. Look closely and you will see skin growing under them. This skin will recede, and the nails will peel over the next couple of days, but if you try to cut them now, you will cause them to bleed a bit. It is better to keep her hands covered to keep her from scratching herself.

An extra finger attached to one or both little fingers is a very common variation of normal. It often runs in families and is more common in African American infants. The extra finger looks like a small sac with a narrow stalk connecting it to the little finger. Rarely does it have a bone in it. Extra fingers are easily removed. In ancient times, extra fingers and toes on both sides were considered a sign of great spirituality.

The Head

The shape of your baby's head depends to some extent on the circumstances of her birth. If she was delivered by Caesarian section and you spent little or no time in labor, her head will be round and symmetrical (B). Delivery through the birth canal molds the head into a more conical shape (A). The bones of the skull are not yet knit together, nature's way of allowing for this shaping, which allows safe delivery. Often there are ridges from the top of the head to the ears in front and in back. The PCP will also check the *fontanels,* popularly called *soft spots,* where the bones are not yet joined. The larger, anterior fontanel is located on the top of the head, midway between the eyes and the ears. A smaller posterior fontanelle is on the back of the head. The anterior may be as big as an inch-and-a-half across or so small as to be barely noticeable. You can gently touch the fontanelles; they are not painful to her.

A newborn's head is covered with a variable amount of hair, ranging from a good, thick mane to near baldness. A fine fuzz, called *lanugo,* may extend onto the forehead. Similar downy hair may coat the arms and back. The lanugo will go away in the next week or two.

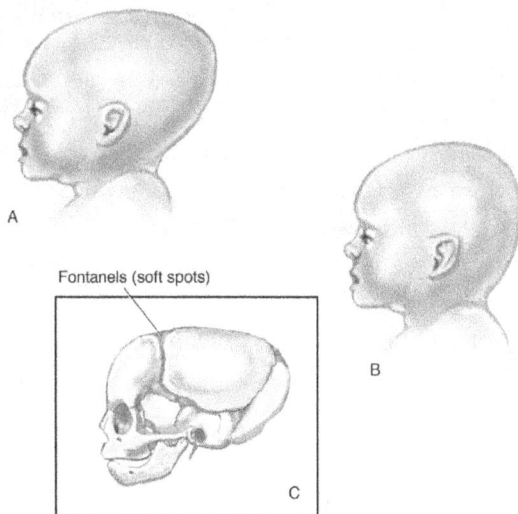

Fontanels (soft spots)

The Ears

Your infant's ears, like her hands, are well-formed miniatures of an adult's. But because of the baby's form, her ears look more prominent than most adult's. Also, her ears will clean themselves. Do not use a cotton swab as it is likely to injure the ear canal. Talk with your PCP about ear care as your baby grows.

Some babies have small skin tags in front of their ears. Most of these tags go away by themselves, but occasionally they must be removed surgically. This is a simple procedure, something you can discuss at leisure with your PCP.

The Eyes

You may have noticed your baby's eyes are closed most of the time. This is partly her response to bright light—remember that she spent the past nine months in a very dark environment—and partly a result of her eyes being swollen. The tissue around the eyes is among the loosest in the body. Pressure on it during the trip through the birth canal causes the swelling. One eye is often more swollen than the other because the pressure is often greater on one side than the other.

This difference in swelling usually leads a new baby to prefer one eye over the other when she is inspired to open her eye(s) and look around. She is most likely to open her eyes when you pick her up and hold her upright, or when you darken the room.

Since her eyes are usually closed and she opens them one at a time, it may take a few visits for the PCP to complete the examination of your baby's eyes. Due to short stays, he may not have a chance to complete the eye exam in the hospital. In that case, your PCP will check closely at your baby's two-week visit, when the swelling is gone. Eventually he will be able to examine the appearance of the outside and inside of her eyes, how they move and focus, and how her pupils react to light.

There may be a small amount of bleeding in the sclera, the white part of the eye. This, too, is from the birth process and usually resolves without any problem.

Your baby's eye color is lighter now than it will be later. You will have to wait for six months to know what the permanent color will be.

There was a time when people thought that newborn infants didn't see very well, but now we know they have good vision. In this part of the physical exam, her PCP will move a bright object slowly past her face and watch her follow it with her eyes. She will follow your face even more eagerly, if you give her the opportunity when she is in a quiet alert state.

The PCP will shine a light in her eyes and observe the pupils. They should be equal in size and get smaller in response to the light. He should be able to see a red reflex in response to the light. The red reflex is light being reflected off the retina, the tissue at the back of the eye that gathers light and holds the specialized nerves needed for sight. You see the same phenomenon when someone's eyes appear red in a flash photo.

Small red spots often appear on the upper eyelids and above the nose. Called *nevi flammeus,* or *stork bites,* they are simply small blood vessels. These spots will recede over the next few weeks without any attention. Interestingly, nevi were considered a sign of royalty in ancient times. Other birth marks may be capillary hemangiomas (small open blood vessels). Hemangiomas usually resolve as well, but may take longer.

The Nose

Newborns have small pug noses with, quite often, tiny white spots. These spots, called *milia,* are small sweat glands that are still being formed. They will come and go for a few weeks.

Both nostrils should be open and, if you listen closely, you can hear air passing through them as your baby breathes.

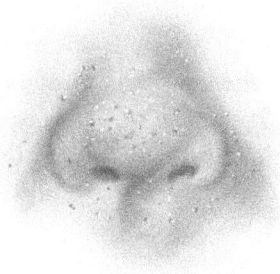

The Mouth

Your baby's mouth is extremely sensitive. If you stroke above, below, or along the lip, she will turn her head in your direction. This is called the *rooting reflex*. You will take advantage of it when you teach her to feed.

Her lips and the inside of her mouth are red, her tongue pink and strong. The connection at the bottom of the tongue will stretch and reshape itself with time. Before people realized that this stretching is a natural development, they thought babies were "tongue-tied" and routinely clipped the connecting tissue. Today, babies are spared that procedure.

Babies generally have no teeth at birth, just little whitish areas on the gums over the spots where teeth are developing. Occasionally, though, a baby arrives with one or two lower teeth already in. If this is the case, your PCP will check, possibly by taking a dental x-ray, to determine whether they are so-called "milk teeth" or true primary teeth. If they are milk teeth, a kind of extra teeth that precede the primary, he may suggest pulling them to ensure the baby won't choke on them when they come out.

Infants' chins are small, perhaps so as not to get in the way of nursing, and often have the same milia as the nose. Clefts, dimples, and the like are common and may or may not persist as the baby grows. The cute ones that make her beautiful will stay!

Examination of the Nervous System

Think of your nervous system as your body's communication system. If your brain says, "Move my right arm," it sends a message down the spinal cord to the nerve that attaches to the muscles of your right shoulder, and your arm moves. Similarly, if your arm is hurt, it uses the same communication system to the brain to say "Ouch," and moves the arm away from the painful stimulus—sometimes quite quickly.

Your nervous system can learn: first you can walk, then run, and then run and bounce a ball at the same time. Your baby has a bunch to learn because she did not need these skills as a fetus—no need to run or walk or even stand—and no gravity to have to deal with. These are all things you will see in her first year, but there is a lot we can observe this week.

Throughout the physical examination, your PCP has been checking the baby's nervous system. He observes your baby's movements and responses to evaluate the health and functioning of her brain, spinal cord, and nerves.

This part of the evaluation addresses one of the biggest worries that many parents express: "will our infant be mentally normal?" Parents' fears about the baby being abnormal often center on a problem that has occurred in their family in the past. These problems fall into three classes: problems that affect intelligence, problems that affect movement, and problems that affect both. I have left space on the next page for you to note any specific fears or family problems you want to discuss with your baby's PCP.

It is impossible to predict in infancy what your child's eventual mental and physical capacities will be. Watching a child's abilities expand and develop is part of the fascination of parenthood. The first neurologic exam detects major problems and evaluates her nervous system as she continues her development.

This part of the exam includes evaluation of both the central and peripheral nervous systems. The central nervous system includes the brain, the cranial nerves, and the spinal cord. The nerves that control movement and sensation form the peripheral nervous system. They are the nerves that feel cold, heat, pain, pressure, touch, and tickling.

The Central Nervous System

As I stated before, a PCP observes nerve function throughout the physical exam. He does this by checking the baby's ability to perceive and respond to stimuli such as touch and sound. These abilities depend on the function of the cranial nerves, the spinal cord, and the brain, and the relationship between them.

There are twelve cranial nerves, which get their name and special status because they come directly out of the brain. They are responsible for the senses with which we perceive the world and for regulating several automatic body functions.

We taste and smell with two of the cranial nerves. Together, these senses prompt us to consume or avoid potential edibles that we encounter. Smell also serves as a means of recognition; your baby knows you, in large part, by your individual smell.

The optic nerve, another cranial nerve, is responsible for sight. It carries impulses from the eye to the brain, where they are processed and interpreted.

Three other nerves control eye opening and eye movement and are frequently immature at birth. If you see your baby's eyes roll up or one eye turn in or out, it is usually due to these nerves' immaturity. The nerves normally mature in four to six months. If your baby's eyes are still rolling up or turning in after the first few months, they will need corrective treatment.

Another cranial nerve controls some muscle movement in the face, but its main responsibility is for sensation. It is well-developed in the newborn, whose face is the part of her body most sensitive to touch, motion, temperature, and pain.

Control of muscles in the face, neck and mouth, and facial expressions resides primarily in three more of the cranial nerves. One of these is located close to the skin, about a half-inch in front of the ear, a location that makes it vulnerable to pressure. Since the head has the body's largest diameter, pressure on it during delivery can easily damage this facial nerve.

An injury to the facial nerve affects the muscles of the cheek and lip. You will notice it most when the baby cries; her cheek and lip on the good side will droop down toward her chin while the damaged side will not move. In the majority of cases, this injury heals by itself and does not interfere with feeding. Only more serious damage to the nerve, which happens infrequently, requires treatment.

The auditory nerve does for hearing what the optic nerve does for sight. It transmits messages from the ear to the brain.

The vagus nerve starts in the brain and extends to the heart, lungs, and abdominal organs. It controls many of the functions that our bodies perform continuously without any thinking on our part, such as heart beat, breathing, and digestion.

The last cranial nerve, essential for sucking, swallowing, and speaking, controls the movement of the tongue. It, too, is well-developed in the newborn.

The second part of the central nervous system, the spinal cord, signals muscles to move, but it depends on the brain for help. In infancy, the brain's control of the spinal cord is not well-developed, so muscle movement is poorly regulated. A slight stimulus, such as a light touch, brings forth a maximal response. The response may repeat; continuing even after the stimulus is gone. One way for you to see this is by rapidly pushing your baby's foot toward the leg and releasing it. The foot may bounce back and forth a few times, a response that would be abnormal in an adult, but is perfectly normal in an infant.

Some of this maximal repetitive response, called *jitteriness,* is normal during the first week, when pathways from the brain to the spinal nerves are still immature. A jittery baby is usually fine. Sometimes, though, a baby is jittery because of a low blood sugar or calcium level, which makes the central nervous system unduly sensitive. If your baby is unusually jittery, your PCP will probably check these values and, if necessary, prescribe sugar or calcium to correct the situation. Within a few days, your baby will be able to regulate her blood sugar and calcium levels by herself and jitteriness will no longer be a concern.

Direct measurement of brain function is difficult at this age. However, as you shall see, the brain functions of thinking, remembering, and learning are quite measurable. Your one-day-old infant can remember stimuli and responses. Even now, she is capable of learning. We see this in a phenomenon known as "extinguishing." The first time a stimulus is presented to her, she will respond to it. The second time, if the stimulus is not painful, she will again respond, but in a slightly smaller way. After a few more repetitions of the stimulus, she will begin to ignore it. She has learned not to respond. Remembering, learning, and extinguishing require a functioning brain. I will discuss it more in relation to other behaviors in the chapters on days two and three.

The Peripheral Nervous System

The peripheral nervous system consists of both sensory and motor nerves that come from the spinal cord and go to muscles and the skin. It functions in two ways: it brings impulses in from the world to the spinal cord and brain, and it carries instructions from the brain and spinal cord to the muscles that move the body. When a sensory nerve is stimulated by pressure, pain, temperature, touch, stretch, or movement, it sends a signal back to the spinal cord, which, in turn, signals a muscle to move. A simple example: you accidentally touch something hot. A sensory nerve in your finger tells the spinal cord it's hot and another nerve signals a muscle to pull away from the source. As an adult with a mature nervous system, you respond quickly, almost instantly.

An infant's peripheral nervous system can receive and respond to the same stimuli, but she will be slower and not as well coordinated in her responses. Stimulating her toe with a pinprick, for example, may cause her to withdraw both legs rather than just the foot that has been pricked. And she may also be slow about doing it. The speed and coordination of her responses will increase as her nervous system matures. It may take a while before you see a faster response to a stimulus to the toe. Since the maturation process moves from the head toward the feet, we see better coordination and smoothness of movement in the head than in the trunk, arms, or legs.

Muscles can move because of a reflex or by intent. Reflexes, such as the familiar knee jerk, are well-developed in newborns, but intentional movement must wait for the circuits to mature in the brain. Those circuits coordinate messages coming in with signals being sent out. Therefore, your newborn baby won't reach out voluntarily for an object she sees and often seems to find things quite by accident, her mouth with her thumb, for example.

The integration that occurs in the early days involves the cranial nerves and enables her to turn at the sound of your voice or follow your face with her eyes. In the weeks and months to come, as you watch your baby grow, you will be able to see how her immature nervous system develops, integrating various functions, which now seem to be operating quite independently of each other. An example of greater maturity is seeing an object and reaching for it.

In the neurologic evaluation, conducted during the physical exam, your PCP has observed your baby's muscle tone, reflexes, intentional movement, cranial nerve activity, and responsiveness to the world around her. If any problem was noted, it may indicate an injury to the nervous system or a systemic disease such as an infection. Injuries often heal by themselves. It is common, for example, for the nerves that control the movement of the arms to be hurt by stretching during delivery. It is frightening to you as a parent to see that one of your baby's arms is weaker than the other, but the trouble is most often temporary and needs no treatment to correct itself.

If your baby has any such injury or problem, your PCP will pay close attention to its progress to determine whether any treatment is needed. Most of the time, however, neurologic signs are just indications of immaturity or variations of normal. Of course, if you have any concerns about how your baby responds to the world, ask your PCP or one of the nurses about it.

Behavioral Development

Your newborn has, for the past several months, experienced and grown accustomed to an environment that is confining, constantly at the same temperature, soft, wet, quiet, and dark. She has been cycling between states of sleep and wakefulness, exercising her limbs and breathing muscles, developing her senses, and smelling and swallowing amniotic fluid. She has had some stimuli to respond to, as all mothers can attest. Loud noises penetrate the uterus and can cause a fetus to change her position. A pregnant mother may cause a change in her baby's movements by her own movement or by eating. Indeed, many women notice a pattern in their baby's activity in response to their activities or environment. And, finally, your newborn has either experienced sustained labor with its rhythmic squeezing or been suddenly expelled by way of Caesarian section.

Her repertoire of behaviors that we shall observe on this first day are those she had in utero. Tomorrow we will explore her reflexes and explain how reflexes combine with behavior states to allow her to adapt to and manipulate this new place. No passive observer, your baby is an active participant in the world from minute one.

This world is a very different place from her world in utero. It is bright, noisy, nonconfining, of many temperatures, and filled with a multitude of sights, sounds, tastes, smells, movement, and change.

Alertness States

As you observe your baby's behavior, you will note her alertness states and her way of moving from one state to another. You will probably conclude that they resemble your own states of being, for they are the same. There are five or six states. The difference between five and six is just a matter of how you define terms and classify activity. For convenience, I will refer to the following five alertness states.

1. Quiet, or nondream sleep: When in the quiet sleep state, an infant has a characteristic brain-wave pattern; breathes slowly, thirty to forty times per minute; and lies very still. A stimulus such as light or noise must be quite intense to disturb the quiet sleep state and cause a response. This is the same state that sleep researchers refer to as deep sleep in adults. Your baby will spend half or more of her first day in deep sleep.

2. Active, or dream sleep: In active sleep, an infant has a brain-wave characteristic of dreaming. Her eyelids remain closed, but her eyes make small movements, as do her arms and legs. The breathing pattern is often faster, forty to sixty breaths per minute, and may be irregular. A less intense stimulus will cause her to respond but not necessarily to awaken. A sleep researcher would call this rapid-eye movement (REM), or dream sleep. Active and quiet sleep states alternate; with babies (depending on age and other factors) often spending as much or more time in active as in quiet sleep.

3. Drowsy: This is the state between quiet alert and sleep. A drowsy baby is relaxed. Her muscle tone is decreased, and she hardly moves her arms and legs. She blinks and yawns but shows no interest in activity surrounding her. When she is in this state, a stimulus frequently produces a startle response or a Moro reflex (more on this later), in which the infant opens her arms as if to give a hug.

4. Quiet alert: This is a waking state. A quiet alert baby breathes regularly, thirty to forty times per minute. She moves her arms and legs only a minimal amount. Her eyes, or eye on the first day, are open and her expression is alert. She responds to stimuli by seeking the source. A baby, in fact all of us, feeds and learns in the quiet alert state.

5. Active alert: Some experts divide this into two states: active alert and crying. For our purposes, we shall consider them as one. When your baby is in this state you will see her actively moving her body, arms, and legs and hear her vocalize. She will have a wide-eyed, alert countenance. This state may vary from minimal activity to a loud crying session and may escalate from mild arm movement to leg bicycling to crying. Active alert or crying babies will often ignore stimuli, and yet will respond to effective soothing techniques.

During this first day, try to observe your baby's various alertness states. You will probably notice she spends most of her time in one of the sleep states. Her excursions into wakefulness do not often go past quiet alert, and last only a short time. Babies that are overstimulated tend to sleep more. The transition from the dark, quiet uterus to the bright, noisy world is hugely stimulating. In fact, if you make your room dark and quiet, your baby may soon come to a quiet alert state and open her eyes. Give her a lot of stimuli on the first day and she may respond by withdrawing into a sleep state.

There is space here to record your impressions of your baby's alertness states. On this first day, just observe what she does without trying to alter it. Watch to see how your baby changes her alertness state all by herself. Notice how she responds to the noises and lights around her and how her response differs in the different alertness states. Observe, too, how long she spends in the various alertness states. Write down the times, especially for the awake states.

You can also begin listing, in the space below, some of your own feelings about your baby in each alertness state. With which are you comfortable? Which not? We will examine later how you can identify your natural parenting instincts, how to use them to interact with your infant, and how your infant will quickly learn to use her wonderful collection of behaviors to respond to you. Right now, it's a big, bright world for both of you to sleep in, if that's what you feel like doing. After all, sleep is one of the five normal alertness states.

	Length of Time	Feelings and Observations
Quiet Sleep		
Active Sleep		

Drowsy		
Quiet Alert		
Active Alert		

Feeding

One of your baby's earliest ways of interacting with you and with the world centers on eating. By now you may have attempted a feeding or two and perhaps she was interested, perhaps not. At this stage it really doesn't matter. Let's consider why.

For the last three months or so, your baby has been swallowing amniotic fluid, practicing breathing movements and, occasionally, sucking her thumb. She has been rehearsing the behaviors she will need for feeding, but hasn't had to coordinate breathing, sucking, and swallowing all at once. Those challenges come at birth and take some time to learn. Over the next three to four days you will see her make great progress with the skills and coordination she needs to feed.

The ideal way for your baby to learn this breathe-suck-swallow process is by feeding with just a small amount of fluid. Your breast adapts to this need by making only a small amount of fluid at first. Called *colostrum*, this liquid is very high in nutrients and low in quantity. It is a beautiful balance: your baby needs a small intake and you have a small output. If you are bottle feeding, you can mimic the low output by letting the baby play with the nipple with the bottle held in an almost horizontal position. That way, gravity does not force milk out of the nipple and the flow is much slower.

In the days preceding delivery, while she is practicing sucking and swallowing, the fetus prepares for birth in yet another way: she stores fluid. An infant is born with ten to fifteen percent extra water in her body to tide her over until she learns to feed. The weight loss that a baby experiences in her first few days is this extra fluid. That's why PCPs expect babies to lose as much as ten percent of their birth weight in the first four or five days.

With knowledge of your baby's behavior states and that she arrived "pre-fed," you can understand her feeding behavior on the first day. First, babies nurse in the quiet alert state, a state in which they spend very little time at this early stage. Second, the amount they eat doesn't matter. You can think of feeding times during the first few days as practice sessions. Expect your infant to be quite irregular and don't be dismayed if she nurses for several minutes one time and just a few seconds the next. Be prepared, too, for her to get out of phase with coordinating breathing, sucking, and swallowing, causing her to gag or spit up. When that happens, just stop feeding and prop her up on your lap or shoulder. She may spit the milk out and be ready to try again.

Most hospitals and birthing centers have lactation consultants who assist the PCPs and nurses who take care of you and your baby. These counselors are specialists in breast and bottle feeding and experts in helping you to understand the process and techniques of feeding your baby. They are an excellent source for any questions or problems concerning feeding.

Breast or Bottle?

A word about breast or bottle feeding is appropriate here. This decision is an easy one for some parents and a difficult one for others. I must start by stating that healthy, full-term infants have two requirements for growth: love and calories. They can get calories from breast or bottle feeding. They can only get love from you.

Breastfeeding does have certain advantages for both the mother and her baby. For the mother, breastfeeding stimulates contractions of the uterus and helps her body regain its pre-pregnant state more rapidly. For the baby, breast milk is uniquely suited to her needs. Its concentration of nutrients adapts precisely to her changing nutritional requirements. Breast milk also provides immune factors that help to protect her from some infectious diseases.

On the practical side, breast milk is the world's original fast food. It is ready instantly, requires no special preparation, and leaves no bottles or measuring cups to be washed.

Some women hesitate to breast feed their infants because they are worried about the time commitment. They plan to return to work or other activities and can't see themselves being available as constantly as they believe successful breastfeeding necessitates. However, breastfeeding doesn't have to be an all-or-none affair. It does, indeed, require commitment on the mother's part, but a minority of mothers breastfeed exclusively. Many breastfeeding mothers use bottles some of the time.

Many experts recommend that you give an occasional bottle to a breastfed baby to accustom her to both sources of food. It also gives Dad a chance to enjoy feeding his child. The bottle can be filled with breast milk that the mom has pumped or with an infant formula. I will explain more about pumping and storing breast milk later. In addition, your lactation consultant or nutritionist will have detailed directions for pumping and storing breast milk.

As far as formulas are concerned, there are many on the market today. They are based on either cow's milk or soy protein and formulated to have a composition similar to breast milk.

To sum up, I think the most important considerations in deciding how to feed your baby are these:

- Breastfeeding has certain specific advantages for both mother and baby.
- Bottle feeding can supply babies with the nutrients they need.
- Choose the method you are comfortable using.
- Whichever way you choose to feed your baby, relax and enjoy feeding her. It should be one of the pleasures of your relationship with her.

Breastfeeding

During the years I have spent examining infants and talking with their parents, I have become convinced that there are as many right ways to breastfeed as there are mothers and babies. The important thing to remember is that you and your baby will be constantly learning from each other and finding the best way for each of you. A couple of guidelines will help you along the way.

First, let your baby stay at the breast for as long or as short a time as she wishes. If it starts to hurt you, switch sides, several times if need be. Doing this enables your nipples to develop toughness, minimizes skin abrasions or cracking, and allows the two of you to try different positions. Even with switching sides, babies often develop a preference for one breast over the other. I don't know why they do this, but they often do. As a rule, this preference only lasts a short time. If it hurts a lot, carefully examine whether she is properly attached. More on that later.

The drawings below illustrate the way most mothers start breastfeeding, which is lying on their sides with the baby facing them. Try putting your bottom arm up around your head and using your top arm to support your baby's head and guide it to your nipple. You may also need to compress your breast away from the baby's nose until she learns to do this herself. As you bring the baby's head toward your breast, brush the side of her mouth gently with the nipple. The rooting reflex will cause her to turn her head toward your nipple. Don't be surprised, though, if she misses or doesn't grasp the nipple. You can help by placing the nipple in her lips as you gently move toward her. She will instinctively begin sucking and start to latch on to your breast.

Having latched on, she may stop after only a few sucks. That's okay. Just relax and repeat the process. She may want to practice latching on a bit. After all, you are both learning how.

There are other positions the lactation consultant will show you that are covered in breastfeeding manuals. If the first position isn't comfortable, you can try another or invent your own. Whatever works for you and your baby is right. Remember to stop nursing and switch breasts if it begins to hurt and the pain increases as feeding progresses. It is important that the baby grasp the entire nipple, including much of the areola (the darker area around the nipple). If baby has only the nipple in her mouth, Mom will bruise and baby will not get any milk.

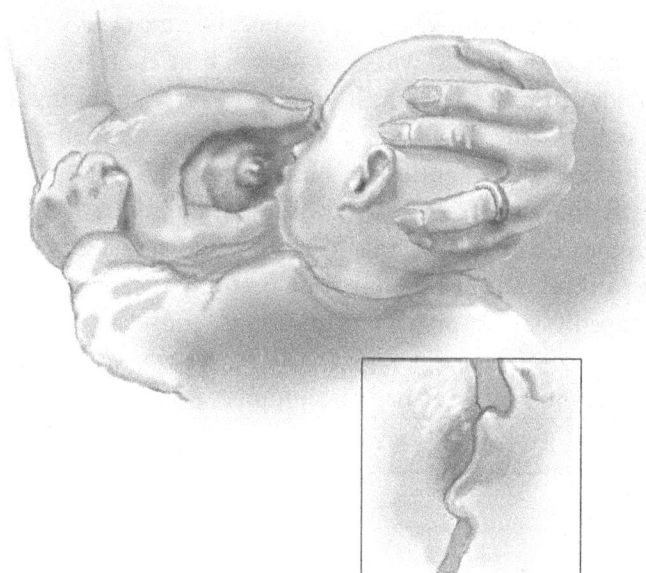

To interrupt your baby's nursing, stroke her head to get her attention and tell her it is time to switch. Then break the seal by pressing on your areola at the corner of her mouth. Gently remove your nipple, lift her head, and make eye contact while you tell her how proud of her you are. Shift your position to the other side, speaking to her and making eye contact to keep her in the quiet alert state and ready to feed from the other breast.

Bottle Feeding

Bottle feeding, like breastfeeding, allows for different positions that offer closeness, skin contact, smell stimuli, and the opportunity for eye contact. The principle here is babies need love and calories to grow, and you can supply both with bottle feeding.

The bottles you will use in the hospital usually contain four ounces of formula. Manufacturers choose this size because they find it impractical to make a smaller size, not because newborns need that much milk. Your baby won't even come close to taking four ounces at a feeding today. I stress this to alert you to a common misconception, that the volume consumed measures success, and urge you to resist that tendency. Your baby will take as much at each feeding as she needs for that practice session. If you try to force more in, often she will spit it back out. Don't be dismayed if that happens—this is a learning process and quantity does not matter.

You will find today that, after short attempts at feeding, your baby becomes drowsy and falls asleep. While she sleeps, you have a chance to think about her and your first day together. It is a good time to record your observations, questions, concerns, and delights.

1. What did you and your baby accomplish today?

2. What did you do that that worked well?

3. What did you do that didn't work well?

4. What questions do you have?

5. What was reassuring to you?

_____
_____
_____
_____
_____
_____
_____
_____

6. What was the most wonderful event of the day?

_____
_____
_____
_____
_____
_____
_____
_____
_____
_____
_____
_____
_____
_____
_____
_____

7. What else do you want to remember?

_____

_____

_____

_____

_____

_____

_____

_____

Now it's your turn to relax. You may need to eat something. A long day, full of excitement, at the hospital or birthing center or even in your home, has a way of making you forget to do some important things, like eating. You may want to rest or to visit with friends and family. This is a day to savor your new experiences and explore your feelings without trying to control or take charge of anything. There will be time for that tomorrow.

DAY TWO
A Day of Exploration

*T*oday, Mom will begin to feel stronger, and both parents are more alert and ready to continue learning about their new infant. He is changing rapidly now, and we will explore these changes with you. You may want to take a few minutes to review the section on the physical exam in Day One to make it easier to recognize what is different today. You also may be going home today or already be home.

Take some time to review your impressions of Day One. Have your recollections of labor and delivery changed overnight? I have left a space for you to note how you feel today and compare your feelings with those of yesterday.

<table>
<tr><td></td></tr>
<tr><td></td></tr>
<tr><td></td></tr>
<tr><td></td></tr>
<tr><td></td></tr>
<tr><td></td></tr>
<tr><td></td></tr>
<tr><td></td></tr>
</table>

You may be feeling confident or scared, excited or flat, up or down, or a mixture of several different moods. There are many reactions to having a baby. I will discuss them in the section on behavior. We will explore, too, your baby's reflexes and expanding behaviors.

You and your baby are ready for more interaction and some new positions for feeding. See some La Leche League materials for help here. Meal times continue to be practice sessions for both of you. He still doesn't need very much to eat.

Hospital or Birthing Center Routines

Before I go into detail about your baby's changes today, let's consider some of the hospital or birthing center routines you will notice on the second day.

Mornings are a busy time. Nurses usually begin their work at 7 a.m. or earlier by making rounds, checking vital signs (temperature, blood pressure, pulse rate, and respiration), and giving medicines. This is a convenient time for you to ask about baby-care classes, lactation consultants, required immunizations, and tests for your baby, and anything else that is on your mind.

Depending on how the nursing service is organized in your center, you and your baby may have the same nurse or two different nurses taking care of you. Both systems work well. The only reason it matters to you is to know where to direct your questions.

Early morning is the time when lab technologists make their rounds to draw blood for tests. There are several common blood tests (some required by the state). Your obstetrician or PCP should have covered these with you.

A technologist may come to draw blood from your baby before you were told a test was ordered. Don't be alarmed if that happens. The need for the test probably appeared during the night, and the technologist reached your room before anyone had a chance to explain the situation to you. This is especially true of bilirubin tests (tests for jaudice levels).

My advice is to allow the testing and later address your questions to your nurse. Here is a place to record the tests and their results.

Test Name	Result

Your PCP will come to see you during the morning. Most come by early, before office hours begin, and this is your best time to ask questions and get the kind of specific information about your child that no book can provide.

Baby-care classes are usually scheduled in the morning as well, so the afternoon is free for visitors.

It sounds like a full schedule and it is. I haven't even mentioned eating meals, showering, and napping, all important parts of your day, as well as caring for and enjoying your baby. You will find this day at least as busy as I have made it sound. You will have so little free time, I urge you to be very possessive of it. Try to define your priorities and keep interruptions to a minimum. I once conducted a survey and found that new mothers receive an average of sixteen telephone calls each day. Silencing or turning off your phone is a viable option! Enjoy all the good wishes, but don't be afraid to keep conversations short, explaining to your callers that you need time to recover and to be with your baby.

Physical Changes

When your baby wakes up, you will need to change his diaper and clean him. At one of the diaper changes, you may want to expand the cleaning into the first bath you give your infant. (The nurses probably gave him his very first bath yesterday.) Many centers have classes on bathing and it would be helpful for you to attend one if you can. For those who don't get to a class, or as a reminder after you go home, I will describe bathing your baby.

Baths

During the first week, sponge baths are recommended to protect the cord from risk of infection. The first step in preparing to bathe your baby is to decide where to do it. Select a stable place where he won't roll over and fall, and where you can reach everything without leaving your baby. Then assemble the following equipment:

- A basin of warm—not hot—water (Test it by feel. It should be comfortable on the inside of your arm.)
- A soft washcloth
- A mild, nondeodorant soap (or baby lotion)
- A receiving blanket
- A clean shirt and diaper

- A soft towel
- An extra blanket
- A deaf ear to the phone

When you have everything ready, undress your baby completely. This is a good time to play as well as clean him. Have a conversation; he will be happy to hear your voice. He will also enjoy the soothing contact and touching during his bath. Dim the light in the room if you want him to open his eyes. I don't guarantee he will, but he is more likely to in soft than in bright light. You will sponge bathe him until the cord comes off.

Using the washcloth, bathe him from head to toe. Rinse the washcloth whenever you need to. Make sure the cloth that cleans the diaper area is not used on other areas.

Rub him gently with the washcloth. You don't need to scrub hard. When you reach the genitals, you can separate the creases to clean them. If your baby is a girl, be sure to wash the genital areas from front to back, as shown in the picture.

Your baby's bath is a convenient time to observe the changes that are taking place in his tiny body.

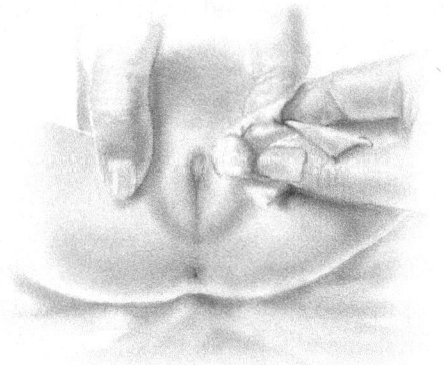

The Head

His head is beginning to round out and lose the elongated shape it acquired during labor and delivery. The fontanelles (soft spots) are easy to feel. If you had fetal monitoring during your labor, your baby may have a small cut on the top of his scalp where the monitor was attached. It should heal in the same way that any small cut in your skin heals. If it starts to look red or swollen, tell your nurse. Those signs could mean an infection is beginning and needs to be treated.

The Eyes

Your baby's eyes likely are quite puffy today. As I explained yesterday, pressure during delivery causes babies' eyes to swell for a couple of days after they are born. It is normal and no cause for concern. The tissue around the eyes swells easily following pressure or trauma.

The Nose

His nose probably looks the same as it did yesterday, although it may have a red spot on it from rubbing. He may also be breathing noisily and sneezing a bit. This means he is continuing to adapt to breathing air. He does not have his first cold or allergies. Air has microscopic particles of pollen and dust in it. To protect itself from them, the body makes mucus. Newborns, who are exposed to these particles for the first time, tend to overdo the mucus secretion for a few days. The noisy breathing and sneezing are their way of clearing out the passages through which the air flows.

If the mucus secretion does not interfere with feeding, it is of no concern. It will taper off in three or four days. If it is bothersome, you can clean it out with some saline nose drops and a bulb syringe. Hold the dropper at the edge of each nostril and put in one drop of the saline. Give it a few seconds to loosen the mucus. Then squeeze the bulb syringe about halfway, place it below, not inside, the nostril, and slowly release it. The suction will pull out any mucus that can be reached. I have included a picture of the process to guide you.

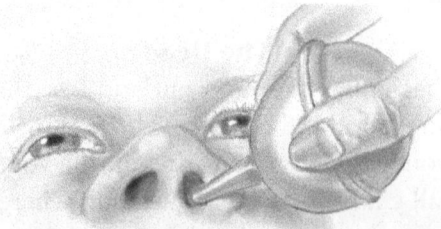

The Chest

His chest is round, and his breathing should be easy and regular today. If you notice any of the retractions I described yesterday, report them to your baby's nurse.

The Abdomen

His belly is still round but slightly flatter than yesterday. His cord is getting darker and should be quite dry. The only care it needs is cleaning with an antibacterial preparation. When you go home, you can also use rubbing alcohol on a cotton swab to dab the cord at diaper changes. It won't sting as there are no pain nerves in the cord. If you are using diapers with a layer of plastic, keep the plastic below the cord. Exposure to air helps the cord dry.

The Skin

The most noticeable changes in your baby are his skin. It appears drier today and may be peeling or cracking, especially in the ankle creases. This change is all part of the process of shedding the intrauterine skin, designed for life in liquid, and acquiring baby skin designed for life in air. It takes a few days to complete the change.

The peeling and cracking may bother you more than it bothers your baby. It is not necessary to do anything about it. You may, if you want to, use a baby lotion or lanolin-based ointment on his skin.

Have you noticed any other changes or differences that leave you wondering? If so, make a note of them and ask your PCP. You will notice that many of these changes become more conspicuous as the day goes on. That is the normal progression for this day of physical transition.

Note any concerns here:

Behavior

Yesterday I introduced your baby's five alertness states. Today I will expand on them and explore the reflexes he has at birth.

During the first day, you could see your infant move from one alertness state to another, although he spent most of his time in one of the sleep states. He will do the same today, but with a bit more time spent in the quiet alert state. He will probably come to this state about eight or ten times and stay there from five minutes to a half hour each time.

Your baby's quiet alert periods are important. They are the times when he will learn, feed, and respond to your messages. On day two, the top priority when he is quiet alert is to practice feeding, but there will also be time to play; in this case, to learn about his reflexes and how they work.

You may find, as you observe your baby's alertness, that he is more alert in a quiet, dim environment than in a bright, noisy one. This seems strange at first, since it is the opposite of how we respond as adults, but it is quite logical for a newborn. Having spent nine months in a quiet, dark place, he finds it normal. Bright, noisy places are new to him, so he tends to withdraw by closing his eyes. Eventually he will get used to the world. He will sleep in the dark and stay awake in the light, but it may be a month or two before he does. We adults say the baby has his nights and days mixed up. He probably thinks we have it backward.

Look at his position while he sleeps. He will tend to keep his legs flexed and his arms flexed and up near his head, whether he is lying on his stomach, side, or back. You should position him on his back to lessen chances of sudden infant death. I do not mention this to frighten you, but to bring up an issue that is in the back of all parents' minds. Although it's impossible to prevent one hundred percent of SIDS cases, studies show the frequency is decreased if infants sleep on their backs and are not exposed to tobacco smoke.

The sleep position reflects his natural muscle tone. Tone means that when a muscle is relaxed, it can either stretch or contract, whichever is needed. You can feel your infant's muscle tone by gently trying to straighten an arm or leg. The muscle tone causes the slight resistance you feel.

Another way to feel muscle tone is by doing an elastic recoil test. Extend an arm or leg by pulling gently on it for about a half minute. When you let go, the arm or leg will recoil back to or past its original position. This may not work when the baby is in a deep sleep and muscles are most relaxed. Lack of an elastic recoil occasionally is due to injury to a nerve or bone. This is unusual, but ask your nurse or PCP if you are concerned.

Reflexes

Reflexes are fun. You are doubtless familiar with the knee jerk: a PCP taps your knee and your leg jumps. You, as an adult, have quite a few reflexes. Your infant has even more. Let's look at some of them to see how they work and what purpose they serve.

Feeding Reflexes

Three reflexes, called *feeding reflexes,* help your baby learn to eat. One of them, the *rooting reflex,* causes him to turn his head and open his mouth when you stroke the side of his lips. You use this reflex in getting him started on your breast or a bottle. A word of caution: if he turns too far, the object that was stroking his lip will touch the other side of his lips and cause him to turn the other way. He may move back and forth rapidly, frustrating himself and his mother. If this happens, move away a bit to stop the stimulus and start over.

The *sucking reflex* follows rooting. To elicit sucking, place your finger in the baby's mouth. He will respond with a sucking movement of his tongue and sucking noises.

You can see how these two reflexes work together as the infant is learning to feed. Rooting causes him to grasp the nipple in his mouth. In turn, the nipple in his mouth stimulates the sucking reflex, which also pulls the nipple fully into his mouth. Having the entire nipple, including the areola, fully positioned in his mouth is a critical factor for minimizing pain to your nipples, and in getting milk to flow.

One other reflex is classed as a feeding reflex. It is a curiosity called the *Babkin reflex*. You stimulate it by pressing on the infant's palms. He responds by opening his mouth and moving his head forward. It's fun to watch, although not of much practical value.

Primitive Reflexes

There is a group of reflexes called *primitive reflexes* because they show up in other mammals, not just human babies, and they disappear in the first year. They seem to be signs of the immaturity of the baby's nervous system. Unlike the feeding reflexes, they have no significant usefulness to the infant. They are adorable, though, and you may want to elicit them just for fun. Or you may want to wait and watch your PCP try them at your baby's first checkup. There are six primitive reflexes: the Moro, grasp, stepping, crossed extensor, trunkal incurvation, and righting reflexes.

To elicit the *Moro*, or startle, reflex, raise the infant's head a couple of inches with the baby on his back and then let it fall backward rapidly into your hand. This is not dangerous to the baby; however, watch a nurse or PCP do it before you try it yourself. The infant will respond with three movements. First, he will move his arms out from his body, then up and toward you and, last, he will spread out his fingers. Below is a picture of the Moro reflex.

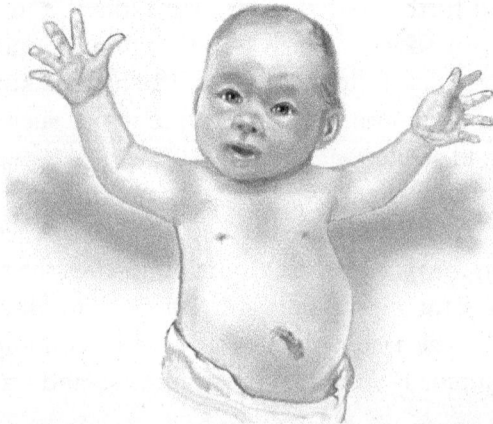

When the baby is asleep, the Moro reflex will still be present, but will be less vigorous. The absence of a Moro reflex could indicate damage to the central nervous system and should be checked out by the physician. A one-sided Moro is usually due to injury to the nerves of the arm or a broken collar bone. The neat thing about the Moro is that it looks like the baby is trying to hug you, and who can resist that?

Feet and hands both have a grasp reflex. You can stimulate this reflex by placing an object against the sole of the foot. The baby will respond by flexing his toes.

With the hand grasp he will continue to hold the object for quite a while. Try it with your finger. You will be surprised at how strong his grasp is. Having your baby grasp your finger tightly is sure to get a smile from you!

The stepping reflex has the baby flexing his legs and looking like he is walking. To stimulate it, hold him upright with his feet touching a flat surface and slowly move him forward. This reflex may take three or four days to develop and may be absent in babies who were born breach.

The crossed extensor reflex depends a lot on muscle tone, so it is decreased when the infant is asleep. You stimulate it by extending one of his legs and pressing on the sole of his foot. He responds by extending the other leg and moving it toward the center line of his body.

The next primitive reflex is truncal incurvation. It, too, may be weak in the first few days and when the baby is sleeping. The stimulus for this reflex is a stroke down the outside of the infant's back. The response is a bending of the trunk toward the side which was stroked.

The last primitive reflex is the righting reflex. When the infant is lying down, he will extend one arm and flex the other. His legs are often exactly the opposite. He will also turn his head toward the extended arm. If you turn his head to the opposite side, he will reverse the arm and leg positions. This is sometimes called the *fencing reflex* because of its similarity to the position of a fencer who is "on guard."

Many babies sleep in this reflex position, whether they are on their backs or abdomens. Interestingly, many adults do also. Do you?

Your PCP tested these reflexes yesterday as part of the examination of the nervous system. You may not have noticed it because they seem to be such an inherent part of infant behavior, but they are some of the things your baby can do that make this time so special. These reflexes are a way of interacting that allows a stimulus followed by a response.

Try some of the reflexes again. This time, instead of concentrating on your baby's responses, pay attention to your own.

1. What did you do?

2. How did you feel?

3. Did you smile or make baby noises?

4. Did you tell your son how neat he is, how much you love him, how proud you are?

You and he are beginning to work together. His response is your stimulus and he will soon be using your response as his stimulus. *Maybe,* he thinks, *the world isn't such a scary place after all.*

Your Feelings

While you are thinking about your responses to your baby, you may also want to examine your own feelings. This applies to mothers and fathers. Parents sometimes experience a down time, called *postpartum blues,* following birthing. Usually it is short-lived and does not interfere with daily life. Sometimes, though, it is enough to make it hard for you to care for your baby. If this is the case, let your PCP know so she can help you.

No one knows with certainty what causes postpartum blues. Mothers experience rapid changes in the amounts of hormones in their bodies after giving birth, changes that make feelings more intense. If this happens to you, we suggest you recognize the situation for what it is: a shift in your hormones that will soon resolve.

Likely, both parents are fatigued from labor and delivery and may be feeling overwhelmed by the change in their lives and the responsibility of being parents.

Another possible cause of postpartum blues is a grief reaction. You may wonder why a parent should grieve after the birth of a normal, healthy infant. The reason centers around the difference between what your mind's eye image of your baby was and what you really have. You may have wished for a girl and gotten a boy, or vice versa. Your grief is for the loss of the mind's eye image. As I mentioned earlier, if your baby has serious medical issues, your feelings will be stronger, and you may want to request grief counseling. I will cover this in detail in the final chapter.

It is important for you to remember that grief for a lost image is perfectly normal and need not interfere with loving the baby you have. In no way does it diminish you as a parent. Give yourself some time to develop a relationship with your baby.

If the feeling persists past a week or seems to be interfering with your ability to function, then some help is indicated. The help can come from your obstetrician or PCP or, if necessary, a psychiatrist or psychologist. Usually, the treatment is brief and effective, but you need to seek it.

Feeding

The first thing to remember about feeding on the dawn of the second day is that the emphasis remains on gaining confidence and experience without worrying about how much your baby takes.

Fluid Needs and Weight Loss

Infants need about two ounces of fluid per day for each pound of their weight. This is much more, proportionally, than adults need because babies have a much larger surface area in relation to body weight than adults do.

Two ounces per pound per day, however, is more than most babies will take in over the first few days. Instead, they use fluid from their bodies to satisfy their requirement. This is normal. As I pointed out yesterday, babies are born with extra fluid in their bodies for just this reason. By the end of the first week, when the fluid reserve has been used up, your baby will be taking more at his feedings. In fact, he will be very good at regulating his fluid balance and letting you know if he needs more.

As babies use their extra bodily fluid during their first few days, they lose weight. This, too, is normal and to be expected. You may remember from yesterday's discussion that newborns' extra fluid accounts for ten to fifteen percent of their birthweight. This allows them to lose up to ten to fifteen percent of their weight with no ill effects. It happens over several days, but the biggest part of the weight loss, between half and three-quarters, will take place today. The table at the end of this chapter will make it easy for you to convert your baby's weight loss in ounces to percent of body weight.

Dehydration

Occasionally a baby will lose more than ten to fifteen percent of his body weight and need to have some extra fluid. Your nurse and PCP will be checking your infant for signs of dehydration: a change in the character of the urine, a dry mouth, a depressed anterior fontanelle, and "tenting" of the skin.

You can monitor these signs of dehydration by doing the following things:

- Keep track of the wet diapers you change. Note especially the color of the urine. It should be pale, not dark yellow.
- Look inside his mouth. It should be wet and glistening.
- Feel the fontanelle when the baby is lying down. It should be flat and resilient.
- Pull gently on some skin over the abdomen with your thumb and forefinger until it has the shape of a tent. When you let go, it should return immediately to its former appearance. If it remains standing up, it is "tenting." Try this test on your baby and yourself today.

If you are uncertain about any of these tests, ask your nurse or PCP to demonstrate for you. These signs of dehydration are not unique to the newborn. They are valid for children and adults as well.

Supplementary (Bottle) Feedings

Dehydration is one of the situations that may necessitate supplementary feedings for a breastfed infant. Babies usually receive additional blood from the placenta at the time of birth. About ten percent of the time, this does not take place and the newborn must use his extra fluid to bring his blood up to the volume he needs, leaving too little to compensate for his low intake in the first few days. Should this happen, your doctor will probably recommend that you give him supplementary water or glucose (sugar) water. It should be given after breastfeeding and limited to one to two ounces. The idea is simply to tide him over until he is ready to take more from the breast. Such supplements rarely interfere with successful breastfeeding.

A few other reasons often lead to considering supplementation for breastfed babies. It's common for parents (or grandparents) to worry about the baby not getting enough. By now, you know not to be concerned about this.

The next reason is jaundice, a topic we shall discuss in detail in the chapter on Day Three. You will see there are some instances of jaundice in which a supplemental formula is helpful, but this is rarely the case in the first two days.

Bottle feeding may be necessary if you take medication that passes into your milk and would be harmful to your baby. Physicians try to avoid these medications or use them for as short a time as possible, but sometimes they are needed. When this happens, you should pump your breasts to stimulate milk production. (All of the information you need about breast pumping is in Day Four.) Your PCP has lists of medications that do and do not interfere with breastfeeding. If you have any concerns about medicines you take, check with your doctor or pharmacist.

Breast problems, such as sore or inverted nipples, or previous breast reduction surgery, may necessitate the use of supplementary feeding.

A nonmedical reason for giving an occasional bottle to a breastfed baby is to give Dad a chance to feed his child.

If you are breastfeeding, this whole discussion of when bottles are necessary or appropriate probably raises some questions in your mind. If you have read up on breastfeeding, you may well have encountered the traditional teaching that supplementation for breastfed babies is unnecessary and may interfere with breastfeeding. Both are true to some extent but, as we have just seen, there are times when exceptions can and should be made. Let's look more closely at the reasoning behind these statements and why making exceptions is okay and ought not be a big emotional issue.

The two reasons usually given for not supplementing a breastfed baby are, first, that an infant uses a different sucking mechanism for breast and bottle and having to learn both is confusing; and, second, that filling the infant with formula decreases the desire to feed and discourages breastfeeding.

The first reason, that it is confusing to learn two ways to suck, presupposes that the newborn's ability to learn is limited. However, you have learned already that your baby arrives with a huge capacity for learning, a capacity that can easily manage different ways of sucking. As a matter of fact, even now he sucks differently on his fingers and your breast. Beyond that, the issue really isn't sucking, which is a reflex, but coordinating sucking, swallowing, and breathing. Babies learn to do this more easily with a low volume of liquid, just what they get from the breast. A bottle delivers a more rapid flow, which may cause the baby to choke and spit up at first. You can minimize the difference by holding the bottle in a horizontal position to slow down the rate of flow. When done this way, breastfed infants usually handle bottle feeding quite nicely.

Concern about overfilling the infant and decreasing the feeding drive is probably more real. All babies need and take very little in the first three days, but they are apt to take more from a bottle than from the breast. Moreover, differences in the composition of formula and breast milk cause formula to stay longer in the baby's stomach. Bottle-fed babies generally settle into a three- to four-hour feeding schedule, while fully breastfed infants feed about every two to three hours. Breastfed babies who receive a lot of supplementation feed less frequently. Since feeding stimulates the breast and promotes milk production, too much supplementation with formula will lead to less stimulation and less production of breast milk. Therefore, if you are breastfeeding, it is better to delay bottles until after the first week. Be reassured that the majority of breastfed infants take bottles at some time and continue to breastfeed quite successfully.

Positions

You are probably feeling a bit stronger today and ready to try some upright feeding positions. The cradle position is the most common one. Hold the baby in front of you, with his head resting in the elbow bend of either your left or right arm. By moving that arm up, you can easily bring the baby's face close to your breast. Your other hand is free to move your breast, stimulating your baby's rooting reflex and helping him latch on. Try this several times on each side and don't be surprised when he shows a preference for one side.

When you use this position, make sure that you have a good, solid back support and are not straining to maintain a sitting position. Both you and your baby should be relaxed and comfortable. You can see each other face to face and make eye contact before, during, and after feeding with a minimum of movement.

An advantage to this position is preserving modesty if you are concerned about interruptions. You can just drape a receiving blanket over the baby while he feeds if you desire.

Colostrum

Colostrum is a pale yellow liquid the breast produces before it makes mature milk. You may have noticed it coming from your breasts before you delivered as well as yesterday and today.

Colostrum differs from breast milk in several ways:

- It is produced in small amounts, a subject already addressed.
- It is loaded with antibodies, which protect the infant from harmful bacteria in the intestine.
- It promotes the growth of intestinal lactobacillus, a friendly kind of bacteria that aids in digestion.
- It has more protein and less fat than milk. Because of its low-fat content, colostrum moves quickly through the intestine, helping your baby clear meconium out of his bowels more efficiently.

This remarkable liquid is precisely designed both to facilitate the transition from fetal life to infancy and provide the baby with aids to survival in the world. Colostrum is a splendid example of nature's fine balance.

Burping

Babies burp because they swallow air as they suck. The air comes from breathing, not from the bottle or breast. To help him get rid of the air after feeding, hold your baby upright on your lap or against your shoulder and gently rub or pat his back. Within a few minutes he probably will burp and possibly spit up too.

Don't worry if your baby doesn't burp after a feeding. It means either that he hasn't swallowed much air, or that the air has passed from his stomach and will appear later as gas. Yes, babies do pass gas.

Back to Bed

When you put your baby down after a feeding, lie him on his back, not his stomach. Spitting and choking are not a problem if you have held him upright for several minutes after feeding, or until he falls asleep. Besides that, cuddling time is special.

The End of Day Two

This has been a big day for all of you, a day of exploration and learning. Tomorrow will include developing routines, a beginning of settling in. For now, relax, enjoy your baby, and pause to realize how much you have accomplished in just two days.

1. What did you and your baby accomplish today?

2. What did you do that worked well?

3. What did you do that didn't work well?

4. What questions did you have?

5. What was reassuring to you?

6. What was the most wonderful event of the day?

7. What else do you want to remember?

Place a photo here.

DAY THREE
Settling in Begins

Overview

Day Three begins with the reality that your baby is here, and here to stay. Often this reality is accompanied by some degree of anxiety. What if she does something you do not understand? Well, this time of settling in builds on the parent-infant interaction that will carry you through the years to come. Both you and your baby are sending and responding to cues.

Today I will explore how those cues can be used: how you can respond to your baby's requests, how you can soothe her when she begins to fuss, how you can begin to adapt the environment to meet both your needs. Today marks a progression of the transitional physical changes observed yesterday. Also, some new things may be happening, including jaundice, a topic I will explore in detail.

Feeding continues to be an issue today. We will explore some of her sucking needs, look at some more positions, and look at the issue of breast and nipple care. Also, today is the time to look at different formulas and reasons to choose a particular type.

Physical Changes

You may look at your baby today and imagine she must be thinking, *this is a rough world*. Her skin has changed since Day Two. It is much drier, with quite a bit of peeling. The ankle creases may even look red. Also, she may have red rubbing marks on her knees, nose, and chin, and cheeks that look irritated. The more you look at them, the more irritated you may feel. It is easy to blame these changes on linens and the like, but the most common cause is the baby herself. She has reached the peak of peeling her fetal skin. With this peak comes a time of maximum sensitivity—the slightest rubbing causes redness. Next week—same sheets, same rubbing, no redness. You can use a baby lotion or a lanolin ointment to soothe her skin today.

The irritation will go away without any lotion or ointment, but this gives you a chance to massage her, producing that close skin contact babies love. Listen to her sounds and watch her alertness state as you massage her with lotion. Special parts are her chest and arms; fold her arms across her chest and gently rock her from side to side and watch her come to a quiet alert state. She enjoys this, and she comes to her learning state when you do it. You have learned a soothing technique, a topic I will dwell on through the rest of this week. You've probably been having so much fun caressing her by now that you have forgotten all about her red, rubbed, peeling skin. It's all right to forget about it because it is a natural and normal process that will resolve on its own.

As you look at her skin, however, she may appear to have a slightly yellow, or *jaundiced*, tone. White babies look suntanned, while pigmented babies may not look jaundiced except in their paler areas (face, chest, abdomen). Most infants have enough jaundice to notice by day three. I will describe this condition in some detail because it is so common and because just about everybody seems to worry about it.

Jaundice is caused by a chemical called *bilirubin*. Every mammal in the world produces bilirubin each day. It's made from the chemical hemoglobin, the substance in red blood cells that carries oxygen from the lungs to other organs. Red blood cells survive only about a hundred days, and when they die, the body converts the hemoglobin to bilirubin. Anything that speeds up red blood cell breakdown can increase the production of bilirubin.

Since bilirubin, as a chemical, does not dissolve in water, it cannot be excreted in urine but must be processed by the liver, which converts bilirubin to bile. The body then uses bile to help digestion.

The balance between the amount of bilirubin made each day and the amount that is excreted determines the amount that will be found in the blood at any given time. So if there is a high production and a low excretion, bilirubin will build up in the blood. In the first few days of life, this imbalance is exactly what is happening.

Let's look at why. While she was a fetus, all her bilirubin was being transported across the placenta into your blood and to your liver for excretion. Since your adult liver is as big as the fetus, it didn't even notice the extra bilirubin. At birth, the baby's liver now has the job of excretion. Efficient excretion requires a maturing process in the liver that takes about three days. This means that bilirubin excretion slows down for the first three days of life.

The process of being born causes red blood cells to break down faster than usual due to normal bruising, so your baby is making more bilirubin than usual. If there is a difference between the mother's blood type and the baby's blood type, the red cells will break down even faster. For example, if the mother has blood type O, she has natural antibodies to both blood types A and B. These antibodies can cross the placenta into the baby along with helpful antibodies such as anti-measles and anti-chickenpox. If the baby has either blood type A or B, the antibodies attack the baby's red blood cells and cause them to break down faster, resulting in more bilirubin being produced. Similar problems can occur with other blood types such as Rh (the positive or negative that comes after O, A, or B). This is the reason your and your baby's blood count and type are often checked at birth. Thus, every baby has an opportunity for jaundice in the first few days and in some, that chance may be increased.

The next question is why be concerned and how much jaundice is too much? The reason for concern relates to the chemistry of bilirubin that makes it dissolve in fat but not water. Chemicals that only dissolve in fat must be carried by blood proteins when they are in the bloodstream. If the amount of bilirubin is greater than the amount of protein to carry it, it will enter the body's fatty tissue. The biggest piece of fatty tissue a human has is the brain. This is the reason for concern about bilirubin. If the bilirubin level gets too high, it can result in brain damage.

The level that begins to be risky for such damage in otherwise healthy full-term infants seems to be over twenty milligrams/deciliter (this will be reported to you as a bilirubin level of twenty). I say "seems to be" because that is the best scientific estimate. In certain circumstances a lower level may be dangerous, and in some instances a higher level may be harmless. If your baby has any of those circumstances, your PCP will be talking with you about them.

Interpretation of bilirubin levels is also time dependent. Normal levels for different ages are known. If the levels remain below these normal values, there is an extremely low chance the bilirubin will get to twenty. Normal values are under four at one day, under eight at two days and under twelve at three or more days. This means that a level of eight on day one would be cause for concern, but on day three would be of no concern at all. If the levels exceed those four, eight, and twelve limits, it does not mean the baby is in danger or that treatment is needed, but only that your PCP will look for a cause (such as blood type differences or infection) and continue to monitor your baby's bilirubin values.

Treatment for bilirubin values that begin to approach the danger level include phototherapy and exchange transfusion. Except in special instances, exchange transfusion is used only if the bilirubin level is significantly higher than twenty. I will not discuss that procedure here because your PCP will discuss it in detail if it is needed for your infant.

The most common treatment for jaundice is phototherapy. Phototherapy is based on the principle that bilirubin is sensitive to a certain blue light that causes the bilirubin to split apart. Once split, the bilirubin can dissolve in water, allowing it to be passed in urine (which is mostly water). This means phototherapy provides an extra way for excretion until the liver gets in gear.

Most doctors do not start phototherapy in healthy babies unless the bilirubin gets over fourteen or so (depending on the infant's age) except in some unusual circumstances. The length of treatment depends on how rapidly the bilirubin decreases. Most stop when the level has reached twelve to thirteen, which usually takes twenty-four to thirty-six hours. After the phototherapy is stopped, we expect a temporary rise in the level that is usually small and does not require restarting phototherapy. We mention this because if your baby becomes jaundiced and needs phototherapy, you may find yourself hanging on every bilirubin value.

Phototherapy may be carried out with the baby in an Isolette (incubator) because the baby should be naked (for maximum skin exposure) and would get cold in an open crib. Some home phototherapy units have provision for crib care and use fiberoptic blankets. These are phototherapy units that fit under the baby's clothes. Your PCP will discuss the various options with you and select the best for your baby's situation.

When phototherapy is done at home, repeat bilirubin levels are collected by visiting nurses and reported to the PCP. These home units do not cause excessive fluid losses and should not interfere with your regular care procedures. Sometimes bilirubin values are measured directly through the skin. Your PCP will discuss this option.

We know phototherapy can be worrisome because of the early hospital discharge of mothers and babies, before the bilirubin reaches its highest level. If the phototherapy must be done in the hospital, being separated from your baby is upsetting. However, by working together with your PCP and the nursing staff, you will find you can continue quite a bit of interaction. Timing in this instance is the key to interaction. The nursery should allow you to be with your baby if you are discharged after twenty-four hours.

Breastfeeding need not be interrupted. If you must miss some feedings, you can pump breast milk for your infant and, as you already know, some bottle feedings will not interfere with continuation of breastfeeding.

I have spent a lot of time on bilirubin because while it is a potential threat to your infant's development if not properly managed, it really turns out to be mostly an emotional issue for parents. It is important for you to understand how jaundice works so you can realize that it is not something you have caused. In certain instances jaundice may even serve a protective role since it is a powerful antioxidant and may protect the baby from some illnesses—another example showing how nothing in the change from fetus to newborn is an accident!

A word here about what is known as "breast milk jaundice" is probably important, even though it's unusual in the first week. The jaundice I have been describing will be highest between days three and five, with the bilirubin slowly (in about two weeks) decreasing to normal adult levels of less than one. Occasionally, in breastfed infants, there is a second rise in the second week that coincides with the production of mature breast milk. This second rise is in the range of eight to twelve. The reasons for this rise are quite complex but probably involve the presence of a certain amino acid that assumes the protective role of bilirubin. Remember, bilirubin has a protective role in elevated but safe ranges for your baby, and therefore decreases bilirubin excretion, resulting in these slightly increased values.

Breast milk jaundice is not a threat to your infant, has not been reported to cause brain damage, and rarely (in the author's experience) gets high enough to require phototherapy. The treatment that works best is to stop breastfeeding for about forty-eight hours, which allows the bilirubin to decrease. Thus, at this stage, PCPs and nurses stop measuring bilirubin and wait for the bilirubin to decrease on its own. Again, I mention this mostly to reassure you that bilirubin is an easily managed medical issue. I know this is easy for us to say and hard for you to do; that's because by now your bond with this infant is intense—a subject I will discuss in the behavior section.

There are physical changes in addition to what you have been seeing. Areas that may look a bit different are the breasts of both boys and girls, and the genital area of girls. The breasts of both boys and girls, especially in breastfed infants, may appear swollen and even have a small discharge of milk. This is in response to the hormones present during pregnancy and in your breast milk. As your hormone levels decrease, so will this breast enlargement. It is important not to squeeze the baby's breasts because this could cause an infection. If the breasts continue to enlarge, appear different in size, or look red, there may be infection that must be treated vigorously. Bring these signs to the attention of your PCP or nurse quickly.

In baby girls, there may be a vaginal discharge. You may have seen this yesterday as white mucus that now appears pink or bloody. Maternal hormones cause a buildup in the baby's uterus that is being discharged. It, like a menstrual period, will stop in three to four days, and not come back for twelve years or so.

If you notice anything else in today's physical exam, write it here in the space provided so you remember to ask about it. Isn't it interesting how well adapted your baby is to make these changes she is experiencing?

1. Add your thoughts here:

Behavioral Changes

Yesterday, I explored reflexes and you saw how the response to one can become the stimulus to the next. We saw how your response to your baby is instinctual. We explored some of your feelings and mentioned the postpartum blues. Today, we will take things a step further and see what your baby can do that is not reflex but learned. We will also explore some more parental feelings termed "bonding" and "attachment," which are a whole lot more fun than the blues.

To start, I want you to believe that your infant can respond to you and you to her, that you can modify her behavior and teach her to modify it herself. I will take this a bit at a time, first concentrating on her behavior.

Behavior is a set of responses to certain environmental stimuli. As adults, many learned attitudes, habits, and the like influence our behavior. Your infant is a clean slate; she comes without attitudes, habits, prejudices, likes, or dislikes. Her behaviors come from her internally perceived feelings, such as hunger, warmth, comfort, pain, and from external stimuli such as temperature, light, and noise. She can learn to respond or not respond to stimuli.

This learning ability is easily demonstrated by the phenomenon called *extinguishing*. To demonstrate extinguishing, wait until your baby is in the quiet alert state, and then provide a stimulus that is not painful and can be repeated at the same intensity. It should have nothing to do with feeding or soothing. Stay away from sight or hearing. Some suggestions are a gentle flick of her toe, a squeeze of her leg, or a puff of air across her face. Watch her response and write it down here. Wait until she returns to the quiet alert state, then repeat the stimulus and note her response. If the stimulus causes her to go to an active alert state, then it is too strong.

Stimulus	Response

Keep repeating this process up to ten times. You will see her response diminish over time, until she makes no response at all to the stimulus. Wait a few hours until she again is in the quiet alert state and repeat the process, using the same stimulus. You will see her extinguish her response even faster. She has learned that a response to that stimulus is not necessary—it offers no reward: no comfort, no cuddling. The important thing is that you have taught your child something and she has learned something. She can learn and you can teach. You and she are interacting.

Next, let us explore some other things she can learn to do. To try hearing, prop up pillows on the bed and when she is in a quiet alert state, sit her against the pillows in a semi-upright position with free movement of her head. Keep the room dim and quiet. Move to her side so she cannot see you and call her name. Initially she may not respond, but keep repeating her name. As soon as she begins to turn her head toward you, move so she can see you and reward her with a cuddle and a kiss, moving close enough so she can smell you and touch you. Try this a few more times; it may take several sessions for her to consistently turn to the sound of your voice. You can tell when she tires and is done with school for the day, because she will start to yawn and slip into the drowsy alert state.

Using vision, place her in the same position, again in the quiet alert state, and face her directly. Look at her eyes and slowly move your head to one side a bit, back to the middle, and then to the other side. She will follow your eyes with her eyes. She may lose you on the first few tries and if she does, move your face back to her line of vision. You will soon learn how fast to move. When she has followed you both ways, give her the same voice stimulation as before, with a cuddle and kiss reward. Again, be sensitive to her attention span and when she gets drowsy, stop the teaching sessions and go for cuddling time.

There is a big difference between the responses of extinguishing and the reinforced interaction. In extinguishing, she learned not to respond because she got nothing in return. In the hearing and visual experience, she will learn to respond because she is getting a pleasant response for her action. She is learning to respond to your actions and you to hers. She is really quite a neat little person, and you are quite neat responsive parents!

You are now experiencing bonding and attachment. There are two separate processes happening. Bonding is largely caused by hormones and is distinct from emotion. It causes you to respond in the first few hours to this baby as just a baby. It may sound cruel, but we could at that time give you someone else's baby and you would respond in the same way—in other words, your first response is nonspecific to the individual. You may have even momentarily wondered, "Is she really mine?"

Attachment comes with the interaction you both have begun. The interaction is not only the exercises, but the cuddling, feeding, holding, and being together. There is no way that anyone could switch babies on you now because you are attaching—a process that is psychological and very specific. She is yours and you are hers.

You may want to take some moments while she sleeps to reflect on your feelings. Maybe some of the down feeling that happened was because you expected attachment to be instantaneous. Now you know it's not, but like all psychological processes (like falling in love), it takes time to develop, to mature, to grow. Smile, you earned it!

Feeding Changes

Today feeding may begin to be easier. You will notice your baby will spend more time feeding. If breastfeeding, you may notice some change in breast firmness and weight: the first signs of milk production. I will talk about how milk is produced today along with exploring your dietary needs. If bottle feeding, today is the day volume will begin to increase. Also, it's the day any intolerance may appear. I will discuss what causes feeding intolerance and why formulas sometimes need to be switched. Finally, today we will look at non-feeding sucking needs and explore the issue of pacifiers.

I have been promising the new mother that she will make breast milk. By now you may begin to have some faith in the promise. Your breasts should begin to feel different today, firmer and heavier, because they are beginning to make breast milk. Questions may occur to you. How do they do this? How do they know how much to make each day? Will they make enough? Too much? Will my baby grow on it? How will I know if she is getting enough? How will I know my baby is getting everything she needs? What about vitamins, iron, or fluoride?

These questions are commonly pondered by breastfeeding mothers on Day Three. Write your questions here so you can ask your baby's PCP, nurse, or lactation consultant today. Leave some room for the responses and don't be surprised if they answer differently. Breastfeeding is not an exact science, and much of the information is anecdotal rather than derived from scientific study. If there is more than one answer, there is more than one right way to approach the situation. You can feel comfortable trying several approaches and finding the one that works best for you.

1. My questions about breastfeeding

The proper name for the breast is mammary gland. I bring this up to remind you that the breast is a gland that produces milk. Just as the salivary glands in our mouths make saliva, the mammary glands make milk. Just as the salivary glands make enough and not too much saliva, so will the breast make enough milk. Just as our salivary glands can be affected by various stimuli to increase or decrease production of saliva, so too can the breast be influenced.

Let's look at the factors that control milk production and see how you can manipulate your environment to make this process as easy as possible. The important factors are:

- Breast health
- Hormonal balance
- Nutrition and fluid balance
- Breast stimulation
- Positive parenting cues
- Stress
- Maternal illness or medication
- Environmental influences

The list may seem overwhelming, but it's not really. Let's look at each factor.

The healthy breast, under the influence of pregnancy hormones and the hormone prolactin (secreted right around birth), causes the milk-producing cells to convert substances in the blood into a secretion called milk. This milk accumulates in storage sacs until there is a stimulus that causes the hormone oxytocin to be produced. Oxytocin causes these sacs to empty into the ducts around the nipple.

If there is no stimulus, the sacs overfill, increasing the pressure in the breast, which decreases blood flow. The decreased blood flow means there is less raw material for the milk cells and they produce less milk. If this situation persists, the cells stop making milk. What is needed for milk production is raw materials, pregnancy hormones, prolactin and oxytocin, and regular breast emptying. If these four are present in a healthy breast, milk will be produced.

The factors of breast size and shape are reflective of the quantity of fat tissue, muscle and ligament support, genetics, and puberty nutritional status; they are not related to glandular function. Problems such as breast reduction surgery, breast trauma or injury, and infection may affect milk production. If these are present, you may need to work more closely than usual with a lactation consultant and your PCP to determine the degree of glandular abnormality. If any of these factors occurred in the past, mention it early, before your baby gets into nutritional difficulty. To summarize, if you have healthy breasts and the hormones of pregnancy, you will make milk.

During breastfeeding, avoid medications that can interfere with milk production or enter the milk and harm the baby. Your PCP will avoid these if possible. If in doubt, ask!

The next big consideration regarding milk production is providing raw materials to your body. These provisions are proteins, carbohydrates, fats, vitamins, minerals, and fluid. Your breast, at peak output, will make fifty or more ounces of twenty-calorie-per-ounce milk. This takes more than forty ounces of water and 1,000 calories per day.

Adjust your intake accordingly. If you do not supply enough calories and nutrients, your body will draw from your stores of calories: first fat and then muscle. You will know this because you will continue to lose weight beyond your pre-pregnancy weight. Plus, you will feel thirstier and hungrier than usual. Your breasts will also draw water from your blood. If your intake of water is too low, early signs of dehydration will appear. The first sign is thirst, and then decreased frequency and amount of urination. If these occur, increase your fluid intake. We usually recommend keeping a glass by your sink and drinking water every time you pass it. If you find your urinary frequency increasing, you are overdoing it a bit.

Breast milk contains calcium, sodium, and potassium. You will get plenty of sodium and potassium from a balanced diet, but you will need to take in extra calcium. If you don't, your body will take what is needed from your bones, not enough to cause them to break, but perhaps enough to cause bone and muscle pain and cause you to be more prone to injury with exercise. Calcium can be obtained from several sources; just make sure you consult your PCP or lactation consultant to determine which source is best for you. Even if you are taking calcium in the form of tablets or milk, you may not be getting enough, especially if you have muscle aches or bone pain (like growing pains at night—remember them?). If you aren't sure, call your PCP or nutritionist.

Eating a well-balanced diet provides protein, fat, and carbohydrates. While you are in the birthing center or hospital, consult with a nutritionist. All centers have them on the staff. They can help you plan how to have a balanced diet that promotes healthy breastfeeding. This is a great time to do it—you won't have time once you get home. Here is some space to write your nutritional questions and jot down the tips you receive.

Questions	Tips

Vitamins also are present in breast milk. You should take your prenatal vitamins to supplement what you normally receive in your diet. While dietary vitamins are fine normally, in your current situation, you need more to supply both you and your milk. A word about mega-vitamins: absolutely avoid this practice; some of the vitamins, especially the fat-soluble ones (A, D, E, K), can be toxic to the baby in large amounts. In this case, more is not better.

The final area to discuss is the emptying process, which is controlled by the hormone oxytocin and by the physical action of sucking. I've already spent a good bit of time on sucking, so let's go to oxytocin. There are several stimuli for increased oxytocin production. These are direct nipple or areola stimulation; a change in temperature, especially warm to cooler; positive visual or auditory stimulation (seeing or hearing your infant); and sexual activity. Factors that decrease oxytocin production are stress and anxiety, epinephrine (adrenaline) production, heavy exercise, decreased fluid intake, and illness. From these lists we can see you want to be calm and well-hydrated before breastfeeding, create an environment that will be free of distractions and other stress-related interruptions, and allow a time for nipple stimulation, preferably using your infant, but either yourself or partner if necessary. I will be discussing these issues in some detail in the days to come.

Today I would like to look at anxiety. Sometimes we seem to become anxious about trying not to be anxious. There is the natural anxiety that comes with all new experiences. It allows us to heighten our awareness, to spend more time in our quiet, alert learning state. As we learn and understand and repeat those things we've learned over and over, new experiences become familiar habits, easy, and don't produce anxiety. For example, I have discussed only a few breastfeeding positions so far. This step-by-step learning allows you to avoid anxiety during this time. You don't need to make much milk, and your baby's extra fluid gives time to learn how to breastfeed. You will be experienced by the time your baby needs to have more milk. So, the anxiety you may feel now will soon diminish. That is yet another reason all this should be thought of as practice right now.

If bottle feeding, you are noticing that she is taking more today. Not only that, but she is spitting up less and choking less. She is beginning to get the hang of feeding. Your concerns about how much may be not very different from those of the breastfeeding parent. The same advice regarding allowing the infant to regulate her intake applies here as well. The greater danger of bottle feeding is over- rather than under-feeding. I will detail this in the days to come. When your baby drifts from quiet alert to drowsy, she is saying, "I've had enough for now."

Another concern is whether the formula is "right" for the baby. Perhaps she doesn't like it. Or is it a different brand from what my friend used? Or is it the same my last baby started on before she had to be switched? Or is it different from what the hospital or birthing center used? Or is it causing loose stools or constipation? There are many questions about formulas on the third day. Let's look at them in the same way by looking at the composition of the various formulas, how these compositions relate to the baby's needs, and how you feel about giving one or another type of formula.

Formulas in the store are generally of two types: those made from cow's milk and those made using soy as the protein source. They contain carbohydrates, fats, minerals, and vitamins designed to mimic breast milk. The components that cause the most intolerance problems on this third day are the type of carbohydrate in the formula and the presence or absence of iron.

Let's deal with iron first because it's easy. The amount of iron added to formulas is very small because it is designed to meet the iron needs of the baby as she grows. In this coming year, she will triple her size and her blood volume; without extra iron she may become anemic by her first birthday. You may have heard that iron can constipate a baby, and or that it causes loose stools. Probably, except in very unusual situations, it does neither. For instance, in one large study, the group of babies fed iron-fortified formula had the same amount of diarrhea and constipation as babies fed iron-free formula.

Therefore, if your baby develops loose stools or constipation on iron-fortified formula, it is most likely not the formula but something else. If the problem is transient, and only lasts a day of two, forget it; if it lasts longer, check with your PCP. If you want to test whether the iron in the formula caused the problem, get both iron-fortified and plain of the same formula brand. Wait until the baby has a normal bowel pattern. Then have someone prepare the formula for the day without telling you whether they used iron-fortified or plain. Do this for at least three days. See if you can guess which was which based on your baby's behavior. If you don't cheat and peek in the garbage, I bet you won't be able to tell.

The other type of intolerance usually relates to the type of carbohydrate found in all mammals' milk: lactose. This intolerance sometimes runs in families. If your baby is lactose intolerant, she will start having very loose stools today. These stools can be tested easily to see if they contain undigested carbohydrate. If so, a change to one of the soy formulas is indicated. This change works because these formulas contain sucrose as the carbohydrate source. Do not expect the baby's stool to change instantly when the formula change is made; it will take her about a day to clear out the previous formula. Usually this problem is transient, and your PCP may suggest you again try regular formula in a month or so. Occasionally babies must stay on a soy formula; that's fine because they will grow normally with either soy-based or milk-based formula.

Finally, a word about sucking and pacifiers. Babies love to suck. They love to learn and love to practice. There is absolutely nothing wrong with using a pacifier. Realize though, like everything else, she will need some time to learn how to use it. It is important not to use a pacifier to replace cuddling time with your baby. As you have seen, her learning is tied to those rewards. You will soon see that decreasing her fussiness and teaching her how to control her own alertness states is similarly connected. So, go ahead and use a pacifier if you wish, but remember it's not a substitute for Mother or Father.

By the way, if you don't want her walking around at age two with her pacifier in her mouth, you must remove it earlier. The time to do this is at about six months to one year of age, when you see her reaching out for objects and moving from bottle to cup. This is her signal that she is exploring the world with her hands, not just her mouth. That is the time to remove the pacifier or decrease it to only bedtime. I guarantee she will not climb out of her crib, get in the car, and drive to the store for a new one. Besides, by then you will be such an expert on interaction that your soothing techniques will help her learn other ways of gaining satisfaction.

This day has been a big one: learning about jaundice, more information on feeding and its scientific basis, and very importantly, learning about how your newborn infant interacts with you and how important you are to each other. Why not reward yourselves with some long looks at each other and a whole bunch of cuddles and hugs?

1. Jot down some notes on how things went today.

2. What did you and your baby accomplish today?

3. What did you do that worked well?

4. What did you do that didn't work well?

5. What questions did you have?

6. What was reassuring to you?

7. What was the most wonderful event of the day?

8. What else do you want to remember?

Weight Loss Charts

Starting Weight		5% Loss		10% Loss		15% Loss	
Lbs.	Ozs.	Lbs.	Ozs.	Lbs.	Ozs.	Lbs.	Ozs.
12	0	11	6	10	13	10	3
11	15	11	5	10	12	10	3
11	14	11	5	10	11	10	2
11	13	11	4	10	11	10	1
11	12	11	3	10	10	10	0
11	11	11	2	10	9	10	0
11	10	11	1	10	8	9	15
11	9	11	0	10	7	9	14
11	8	11	0	10	6	9	12
11	7	10	14	10	5	9	11
11	6	10	13	10	4	9	11
11	5	10	12	10	3	9	10
11	4	10	11	10	2	9	9
11	3	10	10	10	2	9	8
11	2	10	9	10	1	9	8
11	1	10	8	10	0	9	7
11	0	10	8	9	14	9	6

Starting Weight		5% Loss		10% Loss		15% Loss	
Lbs.	Ozs.	Lbs.	Ozs.	Lbs.	Ozs.	Lbs.	Ozs.
10	15	10	7	9	14	9	5
10	14	10	6	9	13	9	4
10	13	10	5	9	12	9	3
10	12	10	4	9	11	9	3
10	11	10	3	9	11	9	2
10	10	10	2	9	10	9	1
10	9	10	2	9	8	9	0
10	8	10	0	9	8	8	15
10	7	9	15	9	7	8	14
10	6	9	14	9	6	8	13
10	5	9	13	9	5	8	12
10	4	9	12	9	4	8	11
10	3	9	11	9	3	8	11
10	2	9	10	9	2	8	10
10	1	9	9	9	2	8	9
10	0	9	8	9	1	8	8

Starting Weight		5% Loss		10% Loss		15% Loss	
Lbs.	Ozs.	Lbs.	Ozs.	Lbs.	Ozs.	Lbs.	Ozs.
9	15	9	8	9	0	8	8
9	14	9	7	8	15	8	7
9	13	9	6	8	14	8	6
9	12	9	5	8	13	8	5
9	11	9	4	8	12	8	4
9	10	9	3	8	11	8	3
9	9	9	2	8	10	8	3
9	8	9	2	8	9	8	2
9	7	9	0	8	8	8	1
9	6	8	15	8	8	8	0
9	5	8	14	8	6	7	15
9	4	8	13	8	5	7	14
9	3	8	12	8	4	7	13
9	2	8	11	8	3	7	12
9	1	8	10	8	3	7	11
9	0	8	9	8	2	7	11

Starting Weight		5% Loss		10% Loss		15% Loss	
Lbs.	Ozs.	Lbs.	Ozs.	Lbs.	Ozs.	Lbs.	Ozs.
8	15	8	8	8	2	7	10
8	14	8	8	8	1	7	9
8	13	8	7	8	0	7	8
8	12	8	6	7	15	7	8
8	11	8	5	7	14	7	7
8	10	8	4	7	12	7	6
8	9	8	3	7	11	7	5
8	8	8	2	7	11	7	4
8	7	8	1	7	10	7	3
8	6	8	0	7	10	7	2
8	5	7	15	7	8	7	1
8	4	7	14	7	7	7	0
8	3	7	13	7	6	7	0
8	2	7	12	7	5	6	15
8	1	7	11	7	4	6	14
8	0	7	10	7	3	6	13

Starting Weight		5% Loss		10% Loss		15% Loss	
Lbs.	Ozs.	Lbs.	Ozs.	Lbs.	Ozs.	Lbs.	Ozs.
7	15	7	10	7	3	6	12
7	14	7	8	7	2	6	11
7	13	7	8	7	2	6	11
7	12	7	6	7	1	6	10
7	11	7	5	7	0	6	9
7	10	7	4	6	14	6	8
7	9	7	3	6	13	6	8
7	8	7	3	6	12	6	6
7	7	7	2	6	11	6	5
7	6	7	1	6	11	6	4
7	5	7	0	6	10	6	3
7	4	6	14	6	8	6	3
7	3	6	13	6	8	6	2
7	2	6	12	6	7	6	1
7	1	6	11	6	6	6	0
7	0	6	11	6	5	6	0

Starting Weight		5% Loss		10% Loss		15% Loss	
Lbs.	Ozs.	Lbs.	Ozs.	Lbs.	Ozs.	Lbs.	Ozs.
6	15	6	10	6	4	5	15
6	14	6	9	6	3	5	14
6	13	6	8	6	3	5	13
6	12	6	8	6	2	5	12
6	11	6	6	6	1	5	11
6	10	6	5	6	0	5	11
6	9	6	4	5	15	5	10
6	8	6	3	5	14	5	8
6	7	6	2	5	13	5	8
6	6	6	2	5	12	5	7
6	5	6	1	5	11	5	6
6	4	6	0	5	10	5	5
6	3	5	14	5	9	5	4
6	2	5	13	5	8	5	3
6	1	5	12	5	8	5	3
6	0	5	11	5	7	5	2

Starting Weight		5% Loss		10% Loss		15% Loss	
Lbs.	Ozs.	Lbs.	Ozs.	Lbs.	Ozs.	Lbs.	Ozs.
5	15	5	11	5	6	5	1
5	14	5	10	5	5	5	0
5	13	5	9	5	4	5	0
5	12	5	8	5	3	4	15
5	11	5	7	5	3	4	14
5	10	5	6	5	2	4	13
5	9	5	5	5	1	4	12
5	8	5	4	5	0	4	11
5	7	5	3	4	15	4	10
5	6	5	2	4	14	4	9
5	5	5	1	4	12	4	8
5	4	5	0	4	11	4	8
5	3	4	15	4	11	4	7
5	2	4	14	4	10	4	6
5	1	4	13	4	9	4	5
5	0	4	12	4	8	4	4

DAY FOUR
The Awakening

Day Three ended, the visitors left, and you said what a good baby he was fifty times, all while thinking to yourself, *Will this baby ever wake up? Is he all right?* Well, he has been spending most of his time in one of the sleep states. However, if you have been keeping a record, you have noticed a steady increase in alertness time. Today, you will see him "wake up" for real. And as he wakes up, you are going to see more vigorous excursions into the active alert state, or even downright crying. We've already learned he doesn't eat or learn well in the sleep states or in the active alert state. He needs to be in his central state: quiet alert. You've been working on soothing techniques, and today you will learn a few and put them to practical use. I will also discuss the process called *centering*.

Today is the peak of many of the physical changes you have been observing. Also, today I will discuss circumcision: the process, the medical thinking behind the practice, and the care of a circumcised baby. I have put this topic here more out of convenience than timing. You may already be home today, with circumcision performed two days ago. Some of you will experience this process in another four days. In either case, follow the story over the next few days as if it were the time of the event.

Today is the day that feeding usually begins to increase in both time and amount. You have been tracking weight loss and today it will be near its maximum (see chart at end of Day Three). If breastfeeding, today may present the problems of breast fullness (sometimes called *engorgement)* and sore nipples.

You may want to pause a few moments and think over the past three days. Your feelings, questions, and concerns are important. Today, if you are home, you may be having a nurse visit your home or going to your PCP's office for a bilirubin and weight check. Give yourself the gift of time to review what has happened, how your baby has changed, what you have learned, and any questions or concerns.

1. Write your thoughts in the comment section.

Now, let's get on with Day Four, an interesting change from the first three days.

Physical Changes

Your baby's skin still looks dry and is peeling, maybe even enough to cause small cracks, especially around his ankles. Today the peeling process may be at its peak. This is a normal, natural process and, again, is more bothersome to you than to your baby. Ignore any comments visitors may make about how dry he looks. It is not the baby that is dry, but simply the peeling process. Remember a key purpose of this book is to record impressions before they fade from memory.

Today you may see a rash that occurs on the body's pressure points (chest, legs, back, face, feet). This rash consists of small (less than a quarter of an inch across) red spots with a pale white center. The spots usually last a few hours and then appear in another location. This rash is called *erythema toxicum*. This terrible name actually means very little. This rash occurs in about a third to half of all babies, starts on the second to fourth day, lasts two to three days, and then disappears. While its cause is unknown, what is known is that it always goes away, needs no special treatment, and is only associated with being a baby. Compare your baby's erythema toxicum to the picture. If it looks different or seems to be persisting in a single location and spreading from there, have your baby's nurse or PCP check it to make sure of the diagnosis. A final point about baby's skin—it probably still looks jaundiced. If necessary, your PCP may continue to measure the bilirubin value.

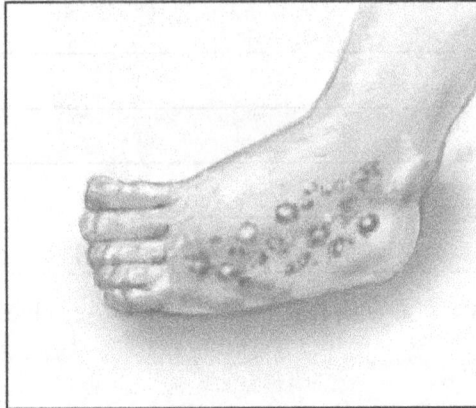

His chest may look flatter today, because it is. This flattening is due to changes in his lung volume. These changes are important and should not interfere with breathing. His breathing rate should remain between thirty and fifty breaths per minute and be quite effortless. If there is a significant change, call your PCP, who will check your baby while he is in a relaxed state.

His abdomen looks flatter, except after eating. His cord is smaller, hard to the touch, and darker in color. It should not have a strong odor. If it still looks moist, remember to keep the diaper (especially the plastic disposables) below the cord so it can be exposed to air for drying.

If you listen to his abdomen, you will hear irregular squeaks and gurgles. These are called *bowel sounds* and are the normal noises made as the intestine moves food along. You may note that today, or perhaps yesterday, stool color, consistency, and frequency changed. As your baby completes clearing meconium from his system, the stool changes to yellow, with a loose, seedy consistency. This is called a *transitional stool*.

If breastfeeding, the stool may look quite loose. If you wonder if it is diarrhea, note whether there is a water ring in the diaper. The difference is that diarrhea stools have a water ring around them in the diaper and they occur unrelated to feeding. You may have noticed he has a bowel movement with or during almost every feeding, which is normal.

A reflex called the *gastro-colic reflex* causes this bowel movement pattern. Basically, filling the stomach causes it to stretch. This stretch stimulates the vagus cranial nerve (remember that from Day One) resulting in a reflex loop that causes the lower intestine (colon) to contract. The contraction produces a bowel movement. This reflex shows how the feeding process in these first few days is also associated with clearing the bowel.

You may also have noticed he turns red in the face, and makes noises and funny facial expressions during his bowel movement. These are all part of the gastro-colic reflex and not a sign of constipation or any other problem. These actions are probably a good sign he is about to have a bowel movement. Do not confuse the gastro-colic reflex with the process called *colic*. Your baby is too young for colic.

His extremities, except for peeling, are much the same. You may note an increase in general muscle tone associated with his increased time in alert states.

His head also looks more rounded, having lost almost all its elongated (molded) shape. This process will continue without any assistance over the next week. You will forget it quickly unless you trace it or photograph it.

Your girl's genitals look the same, but the discharge from her vagina may be pinker or slightly bloody today. She may have some irritation in the diaper area. This is usually not a diaper rash, but a natural accompaniment of the sensitive peeling skin and its exposure to urine, as well as the rubbing from diapers. Some lanolin ointment or cornstarch after changing will help this area during this sensitive transition time. If the area looks especially irritated or has little red spots, bring it to the attention of your PCP or nurse as this could indicate diaper rash.

If your baby is a boy, by now the issue of circumcision has been raised. Circumcision means the removal of the flap of skin called the *foreskin* that surrounds the glans (the sensitive end of the penis). Circumcision started as a ritual, and many religions refer to it. Some practice the ritual shortly after birth and some as a rite of manhood. Because of these factors, there are strong emotional feelings surrounding circumcision. Your decision may be affected by your beliefs.

Medically speaking, there are few indications for a circumcision. They include situations where the foreskin is so tight as to prevent urinating (which is extremely rare) or cause infection. Infection almost always occurs because of poor hygiene. This cause became a reason for routine circumcision in the United States during WWI. Apparently, soldiers with infected penises did not fight well. From there came routine circumcision. With routine circumcision came myths such as locker room teasing (come on dads, have you ever seen this kind of teasing?), increased cancer of the cervix or penis (proven wrong in scientific studies), and the idea it really doesn't hurt the baby (it does).

Let us look at circumcision realistically. First and foremost, it presents a risk/benefit situation. This means if the benefits outweigh the risks, do it. In religious situations, the benefits may be determined to outweigh the risks. One benefit of cirucmcision is a slight decrease in the incidence of urinary tract infection in childhood. Whether this is related to circumcision or to hygiene has not been determined. Another benefit is looking like Dad. This may be important to you as parents now, but is of little importance as your boy grows.

The risks are those of any surgery: bleeding, infection, and damage to the penis. These are unusual occurrences. Another risk is *meatal stenosis,* or damage to the hole at the end of the penis. This problem occurs from diapers rubbing the tip of the penis, and can be helped by using petroleum jelly. The final risk is pain. Anesthesia is available for circumcision, but not commonly used, because the risk of injecting the anesthetic medication may be greater than those of the quick procedure. Using a nipple stuffed with cotton soaked in a fifty percent glucose solution helps during the procedure.

I realize this may be a difficult decision for you. Ask your PCP for more information, especially since circumcision is a rapidly changing area and new information may have become available since the publication of this book.

Circumcision is something that once decided, should be understood. First, the circumcision should not be done before the vitamin K shot takes effect, which is six hours or so. Since the most common complication is vomiting, circumcision should occur at least two hours after a feeding. The actual process takes five or fewer minutes. There are three commonly used procedures: two use well-designed instruments called either the *Mogan clamp* or *Gomco clamp.* These two methods are immediately completed. The third method is the *Plastibell,* which is completed just as quickly, but leaves a plastic ring around the penis. The ring falls off in a few days.

Your PCP and nurses will explain how to care for your infant after circumcision. Basically, care consists of applying a petroleum-based ointment for the first week, coupled with water and mild soap cleaning after stools. Immediately following the circumcision, your son's penis will be wrapped in petroleum-jelly gauze, which a nurse will remove in a few hours while checking the site for bleeding. A bit of oozing with a slight reddish stain on the diaper is common and not a problem. Also, the nurse will check for the first urination for two reasons. First is to assure that urination is occurring normally, and second because some bleeding may occur at this time. You may have heard that babies are more irritable following circumcision, but I have not seen this to be true. Lying him on his side and back and using soothing techniques during diaper changes are good ideas.

Over the next two to three days, you will notice the end of the penis looks quite red. Also, it will appear swollen and may have a yellowish secretion. This swelling and secretion should reach their maximum on the day after circumcision. If the secretion cannot be easily cleaned from the penis or seems to be increasing in quantity, it may indicate infection and you should notify your PCP or nurse. After about two days, the swelling and secretion will decrease, and the end of the penis will begin to look blueish-pink in color (it also, like the hands and feet, is temperature sensitive). This last change is the sign of healing.

Caring for an uncircumcised baby is simple. Just wash his penis as you wash any other part of his body. The skin bridges between the glans and foreskin will disappear on their own. The important thing to know is that the foreskin will not fully retract for quite a while—perhaps a year or more. You do not have to forcibly try to retract it. When it is easily retractable, begin to show your son how to wash his penis just like you show him how to wash his ears. The penis is easier to wash anyway, because at about age one, he'll grab hold of it and won't let go until he is ninety-nine!

We've spent a long time on circumcision, which if you've had a girl, you've been happy to skip. The rest of the physical changes have peaked and now we are heading toward really being in this world. If you've had a boy, give him a close hug. He deserves it—it has been a rough day.

Behavioral Changes

Today is the day you notice your baby spending more time in awake alertness states. He will begin to go quickly from one state to another. In a moment, he will be in dream sleep, skip drowsy, and rapidly progress through quiet alert to active alert and crying. This is a day to learn and practice soothing techniques.

The purpose of all this soothing is to teach him to bring himself to a quiet alert state. He will not achieve this in the first week, but you will see a beginning by the seventh day. Already, you recognize the alertness states and you can watch him move from one to another.

Begin to watch this process even more closely. You already know that learning, responding, and eating occur in the quiet alert state. The concept of being in this state is called *centering*. Centering is the ability to change from one of the sleep states or the active alert state to the quiet alert state. The eventual goal is to have your baby be able to center himself. Right now, he does not know how. Just as feeding started as practice, so shall this process. Just as feeding started with reflexes, so too does centering.

Today, watch how the active alert state evolves. Write down what your baby does. He may change from quiet alert to active movement of his arms and legs to vocalizing with small sucking sounds to an intermittent cry to more crying to a real crying jag. Your impulse to do something during this process is very strong; but for one or two times, just watch it happen. Remember the extinguishing response; he will not cry forever. He will stop and return to another alertness state. It is important to know and recognize your baby's pattern.

1. Write down what you observe.

| |
| |
| |
| |
| |
| |
| |
| |
| |

Some babies are quieter and take a long while to evolve into a wild, active alert state. Others progress more quickly. The majority are in between. Either is okay; it is the progression and your understanding of it that is important, because your soothing responses are going to be in response to your individual baby's needs. This is his time to tell you his needs. This is your time to be aware of your feelings in response to those needs. You will learn to be quick or more intense in your response if he is a rapid changer; and to be slower in your response if he is a slower changer. Either way, you can fit your responses to the needs of your baby and he will fit his responses to you. Write what you have observed without trying to modify the behavior, just as you did with the alertness states on day one.

Now is a good time to reinforce the learning he did yesterday, like turning to the sound of your voice and following your face with his eyes. Don't forget to reward him with your voice and a hug when he does well. Later, you will use some of these learned behaviors as soothing techniques.

The soothing techniques are stimuli for your baby that are designed to catch his attention and bring him back to the quiet alert state. Soothing techniques rely on both his reflexes and his ability to learn. The easiest are his reflex abilities. The principle is if he is a little bit into active alert, it only takes a small stimulus to return to quiet alert. If he is wildly into active alert, it takes a stronger stimulus, or a combination of stimuli, or a combination—plus time.

You have already learned your baby's most mature and sensitive neurological centers are his cranial nerves and reflexes as well as his fetal experience. Therefore, the soothing techniques you will use include both reflexes and environmental and learned responses. The reflexes are those of sucking and grasping. Holding your baby close to you uses the stimuli of warmth and smell. Voice uses the learning you began to work with yesterday. Taste uses the feeding/sucking process. Darkening or brightening the room uses environmental responses.

Let's try some of these soothing techniques. When your baby is getting ready to feed and may just be entering an active alert state, use a pacifier to stimulate first the rooting reflex, then the immediate follow-up of the sucking reflex. Don't worry about his liking or not liking the pacifier, rather observe any change in alertness state. Did he come to quiet alert? How long did it take? How long did he stay there? How did you feel about it? Write these things down for review tomorrow.

Try using some of the other techniques today as he enters the active alert state. For example, elicit the grasp reflex, observe his response, and answer those same questions. You can also pick him up and hold him over your shoulder while gently patting his back as if to burp him. Try not to talk to him while you do this. Another technique is to fold his arms across his chest, as in the picture on the next page, and gently rock him. Or speak to him without touching him, telling him what you want him to do.

Stimulus	Response

Try to do each of these soothing techniques by itself and when your baby is in about the same alertness state. Which did he respond to, which not? Record what seemed to work with your baby. Record how you felt about the various techniques—which seemed logical, which silly? Tomorrow you will work on using these techniques together.

Today, if you have done all these exercises, has been a long one for both of you and your baby. Do not expect a similar response to each of the techniques. The idea is to see which seem to work best now with your baby, others may work later or in combination. Each baby is unique. How you and your baby interact is unique, and we are finding the way you like to respond to each other. Your right way!

Alertness state	Soothing Technique	Observations

Feeding Changes

Today is a real challenge for breastfeeders, and a success day for bottle feeders. Your baby has accomplished the task of coordinating sucking, swallowing, and breathing, and is ready to increase his intake. He will continue to be irregular as to feeding times and quite variable in the quantity of time on the breast from feeding to feeding.

If bottle feeding, your baby may take as much as four ounces in a feeding. He may still spit up some. Also, he may seem anxious to feed. It will seem to take less coaxing today than in the previous days. Still, the whole process is not yet together. While he seems to have developed an interest in feeding, he will continue to be irregular in his feeding times, sometimes going up to eight hours between feeds or as little as two hours at other times.

There is no need to interrupt this pattern or force him into a four-hour schedule. Believe it or not, the four-hour schedule routine comes from some not very well-done research completed at about the turn of the twentieth century. The research, coupled with eight-hour nursing shifts (two feedings/shift), developed into an every four-hour feeding schedule. For now, let your baby feed whenever he wakes up and comes to quiet alert. If he is not very hungry, he won't take much. If he is, he will. After all, now that he is learning all those neat soothing techniques, he might just want to wake up and play!

Breastfeeding mothers may be experiencing significant *engorgement*. Engorgement is uncomfortable and may make it difficult for the baby to grasp both areola and nipple. The tendency may be to grasp only the nipple, which decreases milk output and causes excessive nipple discomfort. Today is a day for special attention to breastfeeding, for now milk is being produced and success is assured. There are some precautions that can be taken to assist you during this "engorgement day."

Engorgement is caused because the glands that produce milk are filling. The ducts that lead from the glands to the areola area of the breast are not yet fully open, so the milk is somewhat blocked. Milk must flow from the glands to the milk sinuses (little sacs) that are behind the areola. Fortunately, nature comes to the rescue by supplying muscle cells near the milk glands that can contract and push the milk from the ducts to the storage sinuses.

These muscles contract in response to the hormone called *oxytocin,* which caused your uterus to contract during labor. Oxytocin is released when your nipples are stimulated. This is known as the *letdown reflex.* This reflex is just that, a reflex. The stimulus of your baby's sucking causes nerves in the areola to send a message to the brain, which sends a message to the pituitary gland to release oxytocin into the bloodstream. The oxytocin acts on muscles in the breasts and uterus, causing them to contract. You feel uterine contractions and breast tingling or contraction about one to three minutes after sucking starts. This reflex causes the milk to flow.

The more often oxytocin is released, the more milk will flow. The more milk flows, the less it backs up in the milk glands and the less engorgement occurs. The less the engorgement, the easier it is for baby to grasp the areola as well as the nipple. The more the areola is grasped, the greater the stimulus to produce oxytocin. You see there is a cycle. The more frequently your baby feeds today, the more rapidly the breast excretes milk, the less the engorgement, the better the grasp, the less the nipple trauma. The less your baby feeds, the less the letdown, the greater the engorgement, the harder to grasp the areola, the more the nipple soreness, the less your baby will feed ... and on and on.

It should be clear that the feeding plan for today is as often as possible, which means every time he is awake. The key amount of time on each breast is at least a minute or two after letdown. Letdown is also influenced by emotions, and there are a lot of those around today. The greatest inhibition is anxiety caused by the fear you will not be able to produce enough milk, or somehow won't succeed in breastfeeding, or your partner won't like that you are breastfeeding, or other life events that may be bothering you. The most important things to remember about today's learning is this: you are engorged because you are producing milk. The letdown will initially be slow because those microscopic ducts must open (it takes a few times to accomplish this, especially if this is your first baby). If you feel your uterus contracting, you have oxytocin, and if you have oxytocin, the reflex is complete and will work better each time it is tried. (And, yes, if you experienced labor—your body makes oxytocin!)

Your emotions are important. Support is what you need right now. If your partner and family are supporting you, great! If not, then use some of the hospital professionals such as feeding counselors, nurses, social workers, lactation consultants, and PCPs. It is also important to discuss your feelings about this issue. Hopefully you began this prior to delivery.

If this is difficult, these professionals can be a great deal of help. Furthermore, there are parent and breastfeeding support groups in almost all communities. Your nurse or PCP should be able to supply names for you. If not, consult sites found on the internet. It is natural to feel scared and anxious. The trick is to avoid feeling anxious about feeling anxious.

Rather, accept these feelings as normal and as you feel them, let your body chemistry happen. Also remember, if you are really worried about your baby "not getting enough," remind yourself of his extra fluid at birth, check his weight chart for percent loss, and supplement some (after breastfeeding) if you want to. Keep stimulating your body to produce the letdown reflex.

Breast pumping and hand expression are good techniques to learn. These are helpful because they will pull milk out of the sinuses around the areola, allowing your baby to get an effective grasp on the breast, thereby minimizing nipple trauma. An electric pump or hand pump can empty your breasts. Both stimulate the nipple and pull the areola into the pumping funnel. Your PCP or lactation consultant should have a breast pump available for your use. Also, most pharmacies have hand pumps for purchase and electric pumps for rent. Ask your nurse to show you how to use both the manual and the electric pumps, even if you do not need to pump yet, because you may need it later. This is a good time to learn how.

Write your feelings about letdown as well as the pump instructions.

Hand expression is another technique that is effective in emptying the sinuses and softening the areola. Also, it is an effective nipple stimulation technique to enhance the let-down reflex. Basically, the technique involves placing your thumb on the top of the areola area and the forefinger of the same hand on the bottom of the areola. Next, slide the two toward the chest (away from the nipple) and squeeze them together when you cannot go further. Do this with them in the up/down and side/side position and repeat several times on each side until the desired softening of the breast is achieved. This may sound difficult, but it really isn't—ask your nurse or the lactation consultant to show you. If you are going to hand express or pump before feeding today, do it to produce only a small amount and start when you see your baby just begin to enter the drowsy state. It is challenging to pump or hand express and soothe a crying baby at the same time. Understanding your baby's alertness patterns is helpful and practical.

Well, up until today, the feeding process has depended mostly on your baby's reflexes and was directed toward his learning to coordinate the process of sucking, swallowing, and breathing. Now nature has provided a reflex for Mom, a reflex that causes milk to be presented in a considerably larger quantity, but not before your baby was ready to handle it.

Today has been an important day, since your baby has begun to awaken, your breast has begun to awaken, working together has begun to take on an active, interactional process rather than a passive or reflex process. There has been a lot to learn and a lot to share. How do you feel today—write down the areas you are comfortable with and the areas that bother you. What seems to be going well? What areas need more practice? Are there questions you want to ask your PCP or your support person or your lactation consultant? If there are, write them down and pick up the phone. If you have questions and don't have a support resource, call your PCP's office for a referral. This also may be an area where friends are helpful.

Write your thoughts for the day.

1. What did you and your baby accomplish today?

2. What did you do that worked well?

3. What did you do that didn't work well?

4. What questions did you have?

5. What was reassuring to you?

6. What was the most wonderful event of the day?

7. What else do you want to remember?

Place a photo (the old-fashioned paper kind) here.

Getting Used to Change

*T*oday is a day to build on the awakening of Day Four. This is a day dedicated to getting used to the changes in your baby and developing confidence in your ability to interact with her. You are moving toward a time of organization, a time where you and your baby can form a more logical routine. Today we will see a resolution of many of the physical changes, some new things occur, and I will discuss how to dress baby for each season.

Behavior assumes a major role now. We will continue investigating the use of soothing techniques and how your baby responds to them. Also, this is a day when your emotions may be at a high point.

Feeding will start to become fun. It has been such a job in the first four days! Today, I will discuss more breastfeeding procedures and breast care. Your baby is approaching a time of organization, so a discussion of scheduling fits well on this day of getting used to change.

Physical Changes
Finally, your baby's peeling skin is resolving and being replaced by silky-smooth baby skin. The scalp clip spot (where a fetal monitor may have been attached during labor) should be well healed. Any bruising from birth is disappearing. She still may have some face scratches from her sharp fingernails, but she is not doing that nearly as much as on day two or so. She has probably learned that scratching herself is not a particularly pleasant experience. Her eyes are no longer swollen, and she is opening both eyes to look

at you. Her breathing is quieter, there is less mucus in her nose, and she is not sneezing as much. She is beginning to get used to her new environment.

If you lie her down to sleep, she naturally goes into a righting reflex. She can curl up if she is cold and stretch out if she is warm. This brings up the issue of dressing babies. How much is right, how much is too much or not enough? There is science to guide us. At five days old, babies are quite capable of controlling their body temperature, but it comes at a caloric cost.

Temperature control relates to calories, as in what we eat. Calories have four purposes: fueling the function of the brain and our internal organs; maintaining our body temperature; fueling activity and movement; and fueling growth. If we don't have enough calories, we first stop growing and second become less able to perform muscle movement tasks (we are tired). Likewise, if we have a high demand for calories in the body needs or the temperature department, our bodies will draw calories allocated to growth and activity. That is how you lose weight—decreased calories and increased movement (exercise) draw from the growth (fat) department. These facts demonstrate the importance of assisting your baby in maintaining her temperature.

How do you help your baby do this? Well, we humans actively produce heat in our bodies all the time. We must constantly get rid of our extra heat. We do that by using the physical measures of conduction, evaporation, convection, and radiation. Conduction is moving heat from a warmer spot to a cooler spot that is in direct contact. This is how you heat a pot on the stove. Evaporation is sweating or why you feel cooler when you step out of a shower. Convection is air blowing across us (the wind-chill factor). Radiation is the transfer of heat from a warmer object to a cooler object. This is how the sun heats the earth and why a fire feels hotter as we get closer. These four processes affect both adults and infants.

Your baby, however, has as some differences from you as an adult. First, her body surface area (the amount of skin that can lose heat) is huge in relation to her mass (the amount that makes heat). Second, she has fewer sweat glands to help evaporative heat loss.

Finally, she is not so good at controlling skin blood flow—remember her mottling.

Pay attention to the four methods of heat loss. In conduction, you would not leave your baby lying in contact with something that is quite cool or quite warm. Evaporation is not a major heat loss problem in your baby because babies have fewer sweat glands. Be aware that this lack also means that on very warm days, she is not able to cool herself as well as adults and older children. Therefore, it's wise to avoid direct outside exposure to the sun (also important because babies sunburn easily). Convection can be an important source of heat loss in a newborn, so don't place her in the direct flow of air from a fan or air conditioner or heat duct.

The most significant method of heat gain or loss is radiation. To change the amount of radiation, consider the distance from the heat source and insulation. In animals, we call insulation fur and in humans, we call insulation clothing, meaning the most significant way to help your baby regulate her temperature is by paying attention to how you dress her.

Let's move from the theoretical to the practical and make some sensible suggestions. First, maintain your house's temperature at a range comfortable for you. Second, count the number of layers of clothing you are comfortable wearing and give the baby one more. For example, on a very hot day where you would like to be naked, give your baby a light shirt and diaper. On a cool day that requires a shirt and sweater, give her three layers. Third, watch how she signals her comfort or need. All curled up in a ball says, "I am cold." Do not look for shivering, because babies don't shiver for the first few months. All stretched out says, "I am warm." These guidelines should serve you well for several months. As you are learning, your observation is a kind of communication with your infant that gives you the correct answer.

Remember, if you are driving in the winter and the car heater is going full blast and you are feeling quite warm, then she is also. Remove a layer of clothing or turn the heater down. I hope this makes sense.

Behavioral Changes

Yesterday, you explored the process of centering and soothing techniques. Today we shall expand on that interaction. You are now familiar with the alertness states. The sleep states still occupy most of your baby's time. Drowsy you've observed, and quiet alert has become your friend. It may seem at this point that active alert is an enemy—not so! Indeed, it is as necessary as sleep. What you are accomplishing with soothing is not abolishing active alert, but helping your baby control it. The movement, vocalization, and activity of the active alert state are important exercise for your baby.

The issue with the active alertness state is its self-accelerating nature. The state tends to feed on itself, starting with activity and vocalization, then crying and air swallowing, with discomfort from stomach distention leading to more crying and more air swallowing, and on and on. Avoiding that cycle is the goal. Even though it is the most difficult to soothe, if your baby has experienced such a state a few times, you have learned she does not stay there forever.

Isn't it fascinating how many cycles your baby has? Basically, that's the way we humans work, because our action causes a feedback that tells us whether to keep going or to change direction.

Today we will combine soothing techniques as your baby begins to increase her active alert state. Reviewing her responses to the soothing techniques you tried yesterday, you may have noticed you felt strong urges to combine some of them, like holding and talking, or holding and rocking, or a pacifier and holding, or holding and talking and walking around or rocking. Today, that is exactly what you shall do.

In the beginning of the active alert state, try a single stimulus; if there is no response, add another. For example, fold her arms across her chest and gently rock her side to side, then add in your voice close to her ear with a *shhhhhhhh* noise. If she comes to quiet alert, give her words and a hug as a reward. Then begin feeding, especially if you are breastfeeding, for frequency remains important today.

Dads especially may have noticed that babies selectively hear higher pitched sounds. Ever wonder why your wife's voice is high and lullabies have higher notes? There is a reason for this. Ever notice how experienced parents often talk to their infant in a high-pitched voice? It's because the baby does not hear some low-pitched sounds. Save those deep sounds for football discussions and use your high baby voice for your daughter during this first month.

Use this process with various soothing techniques: try voice alone, then add holding, then add rocking, and finally a pacifier. Write down what seems to work. Was it changing the room lighting, adding a pacifier, rocking, and singing? Which combinations seem to work? Which does she ignore? Which relate to what level of active alert? In other words, start with what works when she is vocalizing, what works for mild crying, what works for active crying.

Write your thoughts in the table below.

Stimulus 1	Stimulus 2	Stimulus 3	Response

Consider which combinations you are comfortable with, and which not. Remember, you will need to practice this exercise a few times. Just like following your face or turning to your voice, it may take several times for her to learn. Remember to give her a hug and kiss and an "I'm proud of you" award every time she responds. You are developing your own unique methods of parenting your own individual baby!

Also, expect some frustration as you all learn this process. Sometimes she may not seem to respond to any of these soothing techniques. If so, check her for wet or dirty diapers, make sure she is not pinched by some curious tuck of baby clothes, and if not, continue the process. Remember that a bit of crying will not hurt her, and she will eventually stop; when she does, reward her as before. She is learning and so are you.

Now is a time to discover your own soothing techniques. If you think of something, try it! Parents frequently develop their own methods and techniques. As you write your techniques, you will see they are based on your baby's learned behaviors or reflexes. Above all, don't abandon a technique or series of techniques if they don't work at first. Give her some time to learn.

As a new mother, your feelings may be reaching a high intensity today. You feel a mix of elation and frustration at times. Your hormone levels are rapidly changing. You may still be feeling some down times—this applies to Dad, too. You both are beginning to realize that your life has now completely changed dramatically from what it was before. That is true whether this is your first or fifth baby.

Indeed, your life has changed. It is normal and healthy for humans to grieve what has been lost. In this case, what has been lost is your previous lifestyle. Allow this grief reaction to proceed to its conclusion. You may feel shock and denial; you may even awaken one morning forgetting you had a baby! You'll experience some anger and some depression. These may present in interesting ways, like snapping at your partner, a friend, or a well-meaning parent or parent-in-law. Finally, the comfort of resolution will come; yes, your lifestyle has changed, but you need not abandon all you did and liked before. Again, the message with this grief reaction is the same as before: let it happen. If it is interfering with your ability to function, seek professional assistance.

Feeding Changes

For the breastfeeders, yesterday was a transition time. Today will be easier. By now your baby is getting the hang of eating. Your engorgement may still be present, or even just starting—either is okay. Remember, this is not a competition but a process. You may be just starting to make milk, especially if your baby was born a week or two early. If so, just pretend the material discussed on day four is today's material for you.

Frequent feedings continue to be important. Comparing the composition of human milk to that of other mammals, humans fit into the category of frequent feeders. Some mammals, like seals, have high-fat milk and young seals only feed two or three times a day. Humans have low-fat milk and human infants must feed often.

Today you will see your baby come to quiet alert and be ready to feed much more frequently than before. When she does, go ahead and feed her. Frequent and small feedings enhance the number of times you experience the letdown reflex and promote breast emptying. Plus, this gives a maximum chance for your baby to practice her newfound skills.

It is important to realize that ninety percent of the breast's content is emptied in the first five minutes of feeding. So, frequent and short feedings do not deprive her of volume, but rather enhance milk production through frequent emptying and increased oxytocin production with the stimulation of sucking. Now is the time to begin keeping track of which breast you finished feeding on and to start with that one for the next feeding. This is in case she does not completely empty the last breast, and complete emptying is an important factor in increasing milk production and decreasing the potential of breast engorgement and infection. A useful technique is to mark the bra strap of the last breast used.

Breast care is another important topic. Nipples should be kept clean and dry. A hydrous lanolin cream or Vitamin A&D ointment may be rubbed well into the nipples between feedings if the nipples are sore. Exposing the nipples to dry heat from a light bulb or hair dryer will help with toughening and healing. Remember, you are exposing, not cooking; if it feels too hot, stop! If an area of the nipple is sore, it may be due to using the same nursing position repetitively. Changing positions frequently helps prevent nipple soreness and helps your baby get used to change. There are variations of the football or frontal positions that place the baby's mouth at different angles on the nipple. Try using different angles and see what feels best for you.

Bottle-fed babies will be quite vigorous today, perhaps even too much so. They will tend to feed fast and finish a bottle in just a few moments. The tendency is to give a second bottle, which will be consumed just as fast. Vomiting usually follows such a pattern. The important thing to realize is the baby has now developed a vigorous suck and the milk comes easily from the bottle's nipple.

Slowing down the feeding process prevents gulping with a lot of air swallowing and allows time for the closeness that is an important part of feeding. To slow the process, stop feeding every couple of ounces for a burp and a cuddle. This makes feeding more than just putting calories into your baby. Feeding can be made into a part of your interactive time.

Resist the temptation to prop up a bottle for the baby to suck by herself. It is important to stop and examine why you feel the need to do this and begin to work on lifestyle changes.

Bottles, nipples, and preparation equipment should be kept clean. Sterile water in the preparation of formula is unnecessary. The last time your baby was in a sterile environment was the moment before your water broke. Bottles and nipples should be washed thoroughly in a dishwasher or with hot water and soap. Formula may be purchased in ready-to-feed quarts, a liquid concentrate, or powder form. Powder is usually the least expensive.

Each day's formula is easily mixed in the morning, bottles can be prepared with the estimated amount needed, and the whole day's amount stored in the refrigerator. The formula is warmed to room temperature before feeding—be sure to check the temperature by shaking some milk from the bottle onto your inner arm. Any formula remaining in a bottle after a feeding should be discarded.

Well, this has been a day of progress. Physical changes are beginning to wind down and development is becoming an exciting challenge. Finally, she is eating!

Relax as you practice soothing techniques. Don't forget to write your thoughts and impressions.

1. What did you and your baby accomplish today?

2. What did you do that worked well?

3. What did you do that didn't work well?

4. What questions did you have?

5. What was reassuring to you?

6. What was the most wonderful event of the day?

7. What else do you want to remember?

Here is more space for paper photos.

DAY SIX
A Beginning of Organization

Your baby has made such remarkable changes over the last five days. Until today, we have been emphasizing the changes and how you can interact with your baby. Today I'll move from this effort on change to a process of organization. Organization means having a somewhat predictable baby and routine. It does *not* mean rigidity in approach, but rather a confidence in parent-infant interaction. Your baby's behavior is predictable to you and your behavior is predictable to your baby. That does not mean it will never change—it will (he will be a teenager just thirteen years from now), but by learning here in the beginning, you will recognize those changes.

There is not much to comment on regarding physical change today. Much of the adaptation process has occurred. If you have been tracking your baby's weight, you probably noticed little change over the last two days, and perhaps even a small gain today.

Feeding will increase further today. Whether by breast or bottle, your baby will begin *demanding* rather than just *tolerating* feedings. This, we shall see, will afford further opportunity for interaction. By the end of today, you will see the beginnings of regularity. The first part of this week was characterized by irregularity: a good performer one time and poor the next. That is characteristic of your baby as a learner. Today you will see him becoming a more predictable performer!

Physical Changes

As you undress your baby, you will notice much of the peeling and red rubbed spots are resolved. His skin is taking on that smooth, silky, baby-skin feel. Also, his reaction to temperature change, while still present, seems less intense. He will still get some mottling and dusky hands and feet, but less intense and for a shorter time.

When you examine his fingers, you will note the nails appear to be peeling. This is the signal that the skin under them has receded and they may now be cut, filed, or simply peeled. You can now safely keep his nails trimmed to a short and manageable length.

His circumcision should be in the healing stages. The second day is accompanied by a decrease in swelling. There may be a small amount of yellowish material that is easily removed with a soapy cotton swab. If it is stuck or the swelling is increasing, there may be an infection and it should be checked. The end of the penis still looks quite red.

The vaginal discharge in girls may still be present and pinkish in color.

The stool will have changed to a seedy yellow color. It is quite soft but without a water ring on the diaper. It should be getting its particular baby stool smell, which is a sweet smell. It is hard to describe, but not unpleasant and is one of those smells in the world that you will recognize forever.

Finally, his eye swelling is gone, along with much of his light sensitivity. When in quiet alert, he opens his eyes wide. His eyes follow your faces well and he seems quite interested in the world around him. He will stare at a brightly colored object, like a ball, for a little while now. It's a wonder, knowing what you know now, that anyone could have ever thought babies could not see!

If you have any concerns about his physical state today, write them in the space provided. Likely, you will be at home by now, so if your questions bother you, call your PCP.

Behavioral Changes

Today I will introduce the concept of balance. You have been noting the progression from one alertness state to another. You have noted how your baby learns and eats in the quiet alert state, just like the two of you. This state can be thought of as the centered state, and that is balanced by increased activity (active alert) on one side and decreased activity (sleep states) on the other. Balance is achieving coordination between the active and rest states. Just as a pendulum swings, so do your baby's states: activity follows sleep and sleep follows activity. Understanding this flow called "balance" allows you to understand your baby's need to spend time in each alertness state.

You have been concentrating on soothing techniques designed to bring the baby to a quiet alert state. You have seen that sometimes they work and sometimes they do not. Also, you've noted how when asleep, sometimes he is easily aroused, and sometimes he is quite resistant to awakening. Yet, if left alone, he will come to a quiet alert state on his own. This process is evidence of balance between his need to be active and his need to sleep.

When you use soothing techniques to prolong the quiet alert state and they do not work, understand his need for balance and allow him the privilege of entering the state he chooses. Try this and see how long it takes him to return to another state: sleep to alert or alert to sleep. Be patient, and when he returns to the quiet alert state by himself, reward him with your voice, closeness, hugs, and kisses. Congratulate him for having achieved his transition by himself.

Write your observations.

Let him know how much fun it is to be in the quiet alert state without forcing his excursions into activity and sleep. Let him learn his balance and use it. Let him know what a varied wonderful individual he is. Let him experiment and learn. Let him use his alertness states. He will learn how much he enjoys the interaction of quiet alert, where he learns about the world, and is rewarded by eating and hugging, and where he can take in all the sensations outside his own body. Watch his efforts at balancing today. Watch him learn to come back to center. Watch him begin to organize his responses. You can chuckle with him as he misses, for, indeed he will as he learns. Eventually his active alert state will be called running and jumping!

Feeding Changes

By now your baby has learned how to eat. He is good at coordinating sucking, swallowing, and breathing, and eating is becoming a pleasure rather than a task. As this change has occurred, so has his increased need for fluid and calories. He has used up the extra fluid he was born with and is ready to handle two or more ounces per pound per day. Also, he has increased his ability to maintain a quiet alert state long enough to take more at a feeding. All the requirements for successful feeding are now in place. Your milk is in or nearly in, he is ready to take more, and he is alert enough to pay attention to the task at hand.

This is a good time to establish a schedule. Although it won't be necessary later, today keep a feeding schedule in the space provided. Note how long he goes between feedings, how long he spends feeding, and how he reacts before and after. The time just before feeding needs attention now because you want to learn his hunger cues. As an example, substitute your own schedule. You go four to five hours between meals during your day and about twelve hours during your night.

As your baby awakens and comes to the drowsy state, prepare for the next feeding. Decide on position and breast or get the bottle handy and at the right temperature. How long does he spend in drowsy state? See how much time you have for preparation. Also, preparing may mean excusing visitors or finding a quiet place for you and your baby.

As he continues to awaken, change his diaper and begin contact with him. Select a time during the day to include his bath in this process. Try different times to see what works best for both of you. Recognize this time may change in the next few weeks. Use the soothing techniques you have learned like voice, touch, and holding. Take advantage of his ability to see you, hear you, and smell you.

Waking time	Feeding time	Comments

As he comes to quiet alert, settle into your feeding plan. Set up a situation that has minimal distraction from phones, TVs, visitors, etc. Your attention at this time should be focused on your baby. Later, you both will be able to accomplish feeding with distractions around you. For now, reinforce your soothing techniques, get him used to various positions, and see what distracts him from feeding.

Distractions are everywhere. They include various stimuli to our nervous systems: noises, smells, light, and the like that can grab attention, especially if the stimulus is new. Such is the life of your baby: the world is new and filled with distractions. He needs to get used to things gradually. So, for today, minimize the distractions by selecting feeding environments that are as free of distractions as you can make them. Consider this question: do you prefer a candlelight dinner or dinner in front of the TV?

As baby becomes better and better at feeding, introduce distractions one at a time. Introduce them because they are part of your baby's world. Doing this one at a time allows you to notice how he responds. This process will take quite a while, actually years, and it begins now. Notice what your baby can ignore and what bothers him. Remember, he has a tremendous capacity to adapt, so the first TV or tablet stimulus may distract, but later may not even be noticed. After noting what distracts him, you can remove the distraction until later and by using your soothing techniques, bring him back to the feeding alertness state. Remember the extinguishing technique from Day Two? The important thing is to spend a few minutes after each feeding writing your impressions and your plan. There is a lot of opportunity for variability here. This process is fun and gives you the chance to modify your environment for your baby's comfort and learning.

Distraction	Reaction

Taking charge of your environment allows you to try both public and private breastfeeding positions. Since the breast has such sexual connotations in our society, there can be an inherent modesty about breastfeeding. Take advantage of this to establish your own family patterns about breastfeeding.

In private, you may enjoy you, Dad, and baby naked together for skin-to-skin contact and warmth and closeness. If so, arrange these special times. Publicly, you may find yourself at a meeting or gathering with little private area other than a brightly lit, noisy restroom. The meeting setting itself may be a more comfortable environment for you and your baby. Now is the time, in the privacy of your home, to begin learning how to breastfeed in public and what environmental distractions your baby can tolerate.

Spend some time thinking about where you will be going, about the environment and about the distractions you will encounter. To eliminate anxiety about the situation when it happens, prepare for it with practice. You need not be jammed into a difficult situation for which you feel unprepared. You and your baby can be ready for anything, because you have been practicing variability in feeding environments. Remember, at first it may not go well, but with practice it will go smoothly. As with the beginning of feeding on the first day—it's practice and can be quite fun. Don't limit yourselves or your baby; you are both tremendously adaptable with practice.

Breastfeeding in public can be accomplished several ways. Wear a nursing bra that is easily accessible for hooking and unhooking. Next is either a loose-fitting or front-buttoning blouse. With a loose-fitting blouse, simply tuck your baby under the blouse. With a front-opening blouse, cover the baby with a receiving blanket or shawl. Try various ways with your current wardrobe and see what works. One of your early outings with your baby may be a shopping trip to find comfortable clothing for breastfeeding. A fitting room is a good place to try them out. Remember, this practice time will allow both you and your baby to deal with interruptions and distractions without undue anxiety. This is a good time to have a friend along—it is tough to try on clothes while holding and watching your baby.

You have come a long way since that birthing time. Both you and your baby have learned a lot about each other. There is not much now that he can do to surprise or scare you (at least until he is a teenager!). You know his behaviors and he knows yours. Enjoy each other as you explore the tremendous experience of parenting. Go ahead, try something new, something you thought of, and see how you each like it.

Write your thoughts for the day.

1. What did you and your baby accomplish today?

2. What did you do that worked well?

3. What did you do that didn't work well?

4. What questions did you have?

5. What was reassuring to you?

6. What was the most wonderful event of the day?

7. What else do you want to remember?

Here is your photo space.

DAY SEVEN
A Mature Baby

This is the end of the first week. As parents, you have been learning all your new baby's tricks and assisting her through the transition from fetus to newborn. It may be hard to believe that only one week ago she was a fetus, and now she is a person with an emerging personality and a whole bunch of neat behaviors. Also, by now you have realized how well you can communicate: not yet by spoken language, but certainly by the developing language of parents and infants.

There are fewer physical changes now. She may seem bigger than when first born. That feeling may be more symbolic than real, but will soon become the focus of your attention. Also, many fears of abnormalities have disappeared, yet new concerns may be replacing them. I will discuss the signs of illness, the ways you can detect them, and the times to call your PCP.

Behavior is now settling in. That is not to say you have completed learning from each other, but rather you have built a base for that learning to continue. Today, I will finish the topic of balance and propose further areas you can pursue as the weeks go by. Remember this when you teach her to swim, ride a bike, or (yikes!) drive a car.

Finally, she is eating and eating well. In fact, she has now become a regular eating machine. I will emphasize the coordination of the behavior interactions you have been learning and practicing with the feeding techniques you are using. The idea will be to develop a spirit of cooperation in feeding behavior. Neither of you needs to control the other—rather the process is for baby, Dad, and Mom to be sensitive to each other's needs, and to use behavior techniques to enhance the feeding and change the fussing process.

I will wrap up this week with a preview of what is to come. This week has been so laden with change that the future, with slower change and more physical stamina, should be welcomed. The next few months are times of exciting development. The interactions you use will be built on the confidence you gained in this first week. You will be amazed as you look back by how much this week has meant—it is yours and your baby's beginning. So, as we say farewell, I'll give some practical tips for your parenting journey.

Physical Changes

There is little to report since yesterday. As you undress your baby, you notice she is more active, more alert to her surroundings, and more attentive to you. Her skin feels like the soft, smooth baby skin you have been expecting. Her beautiful skin needs only mild soap and water. Baby lotions are safe, and babies do like being massaged. You can try massage with your baby using either a lotion or mild baby oil. The process should be gentle, carried out in a warm place where interruption is at a minimum, and pleasing to you and your baby. If you want to know more about infant massage, use the internet to find an infant massage group near you.

Looking over your daughter, you will note the umbilical cord is dry, shriveled, and brown. It should have no odor. If the skin around the cord looks reddened, or the cord is moist and has an odor, check with your PCP, because these are signs of infection. Soon (or in some cases, already) the cord will separate. There may be some oozing of clear fluid for a day or so when this occurs. If the oozing lasts longer than that or the fluid has an odor, bring this to the attention of your PCP. The remaining *umbilicus,* or belly button, may still protrude some, but in most instances, this will not persist. You do not need to use a belly band. I mentioned this before because they do nothing to prevent an umbilical hernia. However, if this is an important cultural practice for you or your family, know that it causes no harm if kept clean and changed frequently.

You will notice her reflexes are brisker and her muscle tone is increased over what you observed on days one, two, and three. At this time, you can elicit the reflexes rapidly, and some she seems to enjoy. Use the ones she likes for play and forget about the others. Remember, they are signs of an immature nervous system and will disappear. The reflex that remains, in an odd sense, is the righting or fencing reflex. Even adults often like to sleep in that position.

The remaining movement changes you will see in the first year will proceed from her head to her feet, because that is how her nervous system matures. This means she will hold her head up and smile before she reaches for objects. She will roll over and scoot before she sits, and she will crawl before she stands and walks. Your PCP will follow her development with you as parents, and will be far more interested in the pattern of development than in the exact time an event occurs.

His circumcision is now healing well or healed. You will know when to stop using the petroleum jelly by the lack of swelling and the color. The glans and the foreskin area should now both be pink. The area does not look irritated and is not sensitive to touch.

Her vaginal discharge is resolving. If a residual discharge remains, it is hardly noticeable. The labia majora are covering the labia minora more. This is somewhat important to note because they can form small skin bridges if not separated regularly. Simply spread the labia and wipe from front to back using a soft wet cloth as shown in the earlier picture.

Her head is rounding up nicely. Do not worry if she is losing some hair; this is normal. She may look somewhat thin on top for a few weeks. Look around at your friends' children if you are concerned and be reassured by their hair growth.

She is opening her eyes wide and really looking at you, as well as many other things. Take note of the things she focuses on as they may be distractions at feeding times. A word about ear cleaning: do not stick anything into the ears that could damage the eardrum. A soft cloth with warm water, held against the ear for a minute or so, will soften any wax and allow it to be wiped away. Don't be concerned if little comes out with this technique; babies make little ear wax and generally handle it well without assistance.

She may have some sucking blisters on her lips. They look like peeling areas. It again is just the response of her tissues to their new use—eating. Nothing need be done. She will toughen up and these will go away.

Her nasal stuffiness should be less, unless it is winter. A cool mist (not steam) vaporizer or humidifier will help decrease the dust and pollens and therefore the stuffiness. Remember the principles of temperature regulation—you do not need to aim the vaporizer at her. You can continue to use the bulb syringe to clear her nostrils, but only if the stuffiness interferes with feeding. Stuffiness that increases should be brought to your PCP's attention. It is most likely not an allergy, but may be an infection or anatomic abnormality of the nose.

You are now an experienced observer of her breathing patterns, her skin color, the feel of her muscle tone, her responses to a myriad of stimuli, and her alertness. It is these signs, as well as her feeding patterns, that become abnormal in illness. If you see deviations that cannot be explained by the environment, call your PCP. This may occur with some frequency in the beginning, which is natural and normal, and PCPs expect such. What is important is that you know the ranges of normal; you already know these in many ways. Continue to use this manual for a while past day seven as you use the same techniques in the weeks to come.

Your baby has completed her transition from being a fetus to being a newborn. Now, watch her grow!

Behavioral Changes

Your learning about behavior began this week with observation of alertness states, reflexes, and response to stimuli. You learned the important interaction of all of these, how you can influence alertness, and finally how, through the mechanism of balance, your baby can influence her own alertness. You and she are truly communicating. All of this has been accomplished in only one week.

The the immediate future, you will be able to refine the techniques you are learning. As you go through today, note the stimuli that seem to catch her attention. What will bring her to quiet alert? How long does she stay there? What are the signs she has had enough?

To do this, try a fun experiment. Gain her attention by placing your face in front of hers, only about two feet away. Start to open and close your mouth in rhythmic motions. Does she mimic you? Many babies do and almost all will with practice. Her eyes will fix on your motion and follow with great concentration. This is the beginning of her mimicking you—a behavior she will continue for many years to come.

Another thing to try in this same setting is holding your face in front of hers with a smile and slight "yes" nod of movement. She will mimic this also. Then turn your face away. What does she do? Many babies first vocalize gently to get your attention back, then turn away themselves and may cry. She is trying to bring *you* back to the quiet alert state!

By playing with your baby and recording and watching her behaviors, you will come up with many more of these games, often played out as nursery rhymes, that you and your baby can play together. She is learning to trust your behavior and you are learning to trust hers. Believe me, you will need that trust as she grows!

Another few words about the surrounding happenings are necessary. These include visitors, traveling, and siblings. I'll comment first on visitors.

A new baby is a big event for the family. Your friends and neighbors shower you with gifts and good wishes. Everyone wants to hold the baby. Remember, you are in charge, but everyone can enjoy this celebration by using a bit of common sense. One of the fears is infection. The understanding here is that the last time your baby was sterile was the moment before your water broke.

Clean is the word we are looking for here, so insist on clean. People with obvious colds or other infectious problems should come back when they are well. Your baby is quite resistant to many of the illnesses that can be transmitted because your antibodies were transported across the placenta in the last third of pregnancy, however, if you feel better, have people wash their hands.

A greater risk is an over-stimulated, exhausted, irritable, and difficult-to-soothe baby. This quickly leads to the same state in her parents. You now know your baby's cues as to when she has had it for play and learning. Be sensitive to these cues and remember her need for balancing. When she begins showing signs of being tired of the cooing and holding and buzz of activity, excuse yourself and your baby and take her to a place where she can sleep. Doing this will relieve both your own and your baby's stress. This is another area you may want to practice with a few close friends before the big gatherings occur.

Traveling will come up sooner than you think. There again is the worry of infection, but again the same rules apply as for visitors. Another concern is dressing the baby for warmth. Remember the guideline to count the number of layers of clothes you need to be comfortable and give the baby one more. Dress her in layers to account for changes in environment. Safety is another consideration. *Never, never, never* drive without securing her in an approved car seat that is properly installed. A small bump that won't bother you could send her flying.

Airplane travel is safe also. You can board early, and arrangements are easily made for strollers and baby carriers. Check with the airline. Usually, the baby's ears will not bother her if you feed on ascent and avoid feeding on descent. She may cry a bit on descent because this is her way of equalizing her ear pressure. If you get any funny looks during this time, feel free to explain to the uneducated.

What to take along can be a task. Loading your entire house into the car for each trip, as well as scurrying about at the last moment, just causes a lot of stress. I suggest keeping a short trip bag (measured in hours) always packed and a longer trip list available. Keep track of what you use for each and it will become simple. You can add or subtract to your list to fit your individual needs or location of travel and season.

Siblings can be quite a challenge at the time of a new baby's homecoming. Most parents have spent time preparing the child for the arrival of the new sister or brother. Whether you have or not, you can be sure the sibling will not like this intrusion into his exclusive rights. At first there will be a good bit of curiosity, of "I want to hold," "I want to feed," and the like. The child's age should be your guide to the degree of supervision necessary here, but some is always indicated as any new activity requires supervision. Next may come some regression of behavior like wanting to be held more, baby talk, loss of toilet training, needing a bottle again, waking up at night, and the like. The message here is competition for your affection.

The fear is that Mom and Dad will not have enough love for two or three, so I'll become a baby and secure my position. There is other complex psychology going on at this time, but the basic issue is fear of losing the parent to this new baby. What to do? The best advice I have encountered is to show by action that the fear is not true. To do this, set up special time for each parent alone and both parents together to spend time with the older child.

This special time is non-interrupted time to read, play, watch TV, play games, or whatever your child likes. Plan it for a time when the baby is usually asleep. By writing notes on the baby's schedule earlier, you know when sleep times usually occur. If the baby awakens, try to finish the activity with the older child before tending to the baby. If the baby cries some, that is okay; you know how to soothe her, and some of the time she can soothe herself.

If the interruption becomes too regular, examine what in the environment is the trigger; is it timing, noise, or some other distraction? During that time with your older child, use the same techniques of praise for age appropriate activity—he will soon learn he doesn't need to be a baby to get your attention. If this technique does not work over a few months' time, or if regressive behavior persists, be sure to discuss this with your PCP. Don't worry, for it is rare for it to last long and when you realize what is happening, it can even be quite amusing.

This week has been so exciting. The techniques you have learned allow you to understand your baby. They provide you the confidence of continued change of interactions that work for you, as you know you can abandon those techniques that don't work as well, and practice those that do. You can tell your baby what you like, and she can tell you what she likes.

Feeding Changes

She can eat! She has learned how and so have you. Breastfed babies latch on easily and stay awhile, often ten minutes or longer. Bottle-fed babies are now taking four or more ounces per feeding. Feeding is beginning to be a mutual pleasure for both baby and parents.

One interesting thing is your baby already knows when to stop eating. She does not continue until she is so full that she overflows and spits up. How does she know this? You have probably guessed— it is a cyclic reflex. As her stomach fills, a nervous stimulation causes her to produce a hormone that tells her to stop eating for now until she is hungry again. We call this the feast-fast cycle. Adults have the same reflex, but unfortunately sometimes ignore it and keep on going. However, when she says stop, you can be comfortable she has had enough.

This is a day to increase the organizational skills you worked on yesterday. Continue to pay attention to distracting factors in the environment and continue trying different techniques to practice for the time you will need them.

If breastfeeding, your milk is changing from colostrum to mature breast milk. The quantity has increased, and you may even be leaking some. The engorgement is gone, now replaced by a feeling of fullness as feeding time approaches. Be sure to watch yourself for mild signs of dehydration so you can keep your fluid intake high enough. If you are feeling thirsty or urinating less frequently than in your pre-pregnant state, you may be falling behind in the fluid department.

Nipple soreness may not have disappeared completely. If it is getting worse, meeting with a lactation consultant is a must. Almost all breastfeeding groups or PCP offices have support personel available by phone. They may even have volunteers who will see you free of charge. They are generally very helpful. Be cautious of anyone who tries to sell breastfeeding as the only way to safely feed a baby. Although I advocate and support breastfeeding, I also realize it is not appropriate for everyone. Your PCP's office should also be able to assist in this situation.

If this is your first baby, this has been one of the most amazing weeks you have ever spent in your whole life. If this is your second or third baby, you are marveling at how different each child is. In one short week, you have learned to communicate with your baby. You can and do respond to each other. You are in charge. You know what to do. You are parents and child.

CONGRATULATIONS!

THE HARD CHAPTER

If your baby is ill, has died, or suffers from a serious abnormality, you are experiencing the worst event you may face in your whole life. You have my greatest sympathy. Your loss has raised the unanswerable question, "If only I had ...". You will fill that blank with many different things in the days, weeks, and even years to come. Sometimes there is an answer, but all too often there is none.

Your grief is intense, affecting every aspect of your day and night. Indeed, as you move forward, you will find that many friends and relatives do not know what to say or do in response to your loss. Often, they say things that increase the hurt. They do not understand the depth and pain of your grief. Some stop seeing you because they don't know what to say or find they cannot say anything. Sometimes people say things like, "You are young and can have others." However, no other replaces *this* baby, and worse, it can feel like their platitude implies that if you keep trying, maybe you will get it right. Or, "Things were really bad; it's better this way," but it is never better that your baby died. They don't say these things to hurt you, but rather because they don't know what else to say.

Let me say what they cannot: your baby is a real person whose life was shortened. Not to grieve his life is to negate his existence. He will always be with you, just like your parent, sibling, or spouse. Your grief is real, and I feel for you. To trivialize your feelings negates the reality of your infant.

I will speak briefly about your grief and the processes of grieving, but with a word of caution. Please, do not walk this journey by yourself. There are excellent resources available to assist you. Some of these are professional and some are support groups. Seek help, because your grief is going to be deep and intense, and it may be associated with serious consequences.

What makes this grief different? Normal grief is a gift that allows us to tolerate loss of those we do not know with ease, and to heal from the loss of those close to us. Normal grief has five stages: shock, denial, anger, depression, and resolution. Dr. Elizabeth Kubler-Ross has written excellent books on the process that allows us to move forward with our lives after the loss of someone close to us. Often either anger or depression dominates the process, but they usually are not life-consuming. The usual grieving process enters resolution between six months and one year after the loss.

I will briefly summarize the grief stages:

- Shock is the "Oh my God, what happened?" phase. It is usually very brief.
- Denial is the "This is not really happening," or "You must be wrong," phase and is also usually quite brief.
- Anger is aimed at others who we could blame for the situation. It may be a person ... the other driver; an object ... if only he had stopped smoking; or an event ... I told her not to swim there. Anger usually lasts longer than either shock or denial, and may cause adverse behavior on your part.
- Depression is a longer phase of grieving. It includes profound sadness and loneliness, often characterized by crying, lack of sleep, loss of appetite, and other similar behaviors. If depression lasts longer than six months or interferes significantly with a person's ability to carry out activities of daily living, professional consultation is essential.
- Resolution is the final phase of grief. Here, the grieving individual creates a memorial to the lost person. The memorial is usually something that was special to the deceased person, like art, music, a garden, or a special photo arrangement. This phase brings peace to the grieving person and allows them to move forward in their life.

Grief over the loss of your own child, whether due to a stillbirth, illness, congenital malformation, sudden infant death, accident, or other cause, is quite different. The same five phases exist, but the anger and depression are intensified. The anger or depression phase often arrests the grief reaction, keeping you from moving forward and preventing resolution.

What is the source of the grieving parent's anger and how is the anger handled? The unspeakable truth is that they are angry at themselves. As humans, we subconsciously believe a woman is less complete if she cannot birth a healthy infant, and a man is less complete if he cannot father a healthy infant. To further complicate the situation, each partner may subconsciously think there is something wrong with the other. Psychologically speaking, humans don't deal well with being angry at themselves. Therefore, they use defense mechanisms to deal with their feelings.

Defense mechanisms are internal thought processes that help us maintain sanity in threatening situations.

You may have heard of some of these, like denial and projection. They are called defense mechanisms because they help us deal with difficult times.

Some of the common ones include:

- **Denial:** An event did not really happen the way they said it did. "I really did not drink that much before I drove home."
- **Projection:** It is not my fault; someone else caused it. "It was the doctor's (hospital's, nurse's, etc.) fault and I am going to sue them (anger)."
- **Reaction Formation:** Converting a sad event into a falsely acceptable event. "It is a good thing Sam died, because we were not able to care for him."
- **Displacement:** Putting a new object in place of the loss. "We are young, and we will change doctors and have a healthy baby."

There are others, but all of these are temporary and require ongoing subconscious energy to sustain. That is a big part of the reason it is necessary to get assistance during this most difficult time.

Another reason for seeking assistance is the research concerning those who do not. Rates of divorce, suicide, addictive behavior, and violence are significantly greater in couples who suffer a loss and don't get assistance in dealing with that loss.

So, where do we get help? Unfortunately, family and friends are not usually equipped to assist in this process. The reason they don't know what to do is because they have not experienced a similar loss, nor had professional training. In the past, before the 1930s or so, infant death was common enough to be a family event, and many friends and family had "been there," were able to appreciate the loss, and had the ability to help. Today, we often must seek assistance elsewhere.

Fortunately, there are groups that have specific training in this difficult area. Nationally, the Tears Foundation (253.200.0944, www.thetearsfoundation.org) is dedicated to this problem. The foundation has chapters all over the US that provide support in many ways. Churches recognize this need and many offer counseling services or support through an organization called The Stephen Ministry, with over 6,000 chapters nationally. The volunteer individuals in this ministry are trained to deal with grief and loss. There are many psychological and psychiatric counseling services available, both private practices and through organizations that are equipped to help. Hospice Organizations throughout the country have expanded services to assist those who have suffered such losses as well, often in professionally facilitated groups of parents who have experienced similar situations. Finally, PCPs are experienced in this area, and hospitals and birthing centers have trained grief counselors.

In my own intensive newborn care practice, every parent I saw was deeply affected when a baby was very ill or died. I will close with my prayers for you and your child and my hopes that you seek and find the support you need.

ABOUT THE AUTHOR

Dr. Frank Bowen became a neonatologist after completing his pediatric residency at Letterman Hospital and his fellowship at the District of Columbia National Children's Hospital. This training in managing sick or premature infants led him to leading Newborn Services at Willian Beaumont Army Medical Center, Columbus Children's Hospital, and Pennsylvania Hospital in Philadelphia. Newborn Pediatrics at that time was a teaching service within the University of Pennsylvania. Also, he found himself managing the well infants (about 4,000 per year). This stimulated his curiosity about the transition from fetal to newborn life and began the embryonic development of this book.

Dr. Bowen has always been a scientist, and during his career, became a member of the American Pediatric Association, National Perinatal Association, and American Academy of Pediatrics, as well as publishing several scientific articles. His career track in managing sick infants changed in the late 1990s, when he became a consultant and subsequently medial director of Volunteers in Medicine on Hilton Head Island, a free clinic that sees over 30,000 patients per year. From there, he joined the board of the Hospice Care of the Lowcountry and participated in the facilitation of parents who had lost infants. He was hugely impressed with how little the general population knows about how their bodies work, and how much those who are trained must share. Hence the background for this "User's Manual."

Mothers now leave the hospital often at less than a day after birth. Baby and child care books are valuable sources of information, but often are light on the fetal to newborn transition. Specialization in medicine has, in many cases, removed the practicing child care provider from the hospital care of the newly born infant. However, when we buy an automobile, refrigerator, or any other gadget, we get a user's manual, often of more than a hundred pages. Not so when people "get" a new baby, an occurrence that happens about four million times a year in the United States alone.

Dr. Bowen has a passion for sharing knowledge, hopefully in ways that are useful to the receiver. He invites your comments and thoughts, because the vast majority of what he learned about babies and mothers came from parents like you. Finally, he is grateful to those researchers and observers who have written scientifically about what they have observed, including Dr. T. Berry Brazelton, Marshal Klaus, John Kennell, Lu Lubchenco, and a good friend, Ben Spock. The names could go on and on. In the midst of the excitement of great discoveries in the management of sick infants in the 1970s and 1980s, these and others saw the power and importance of the well infant-parent bond that is critical both to our individual development and to our society as a whole.

I N D E X

www.ingramcontent.com/pod-product-compliance
Lightning Source LLC
LaVergne TN
LVHW091217080426
835509LV00009B/1038